PRAISE FOR *THE DEAF BABY INSTRUCTION MANUAL*

"Every parent of a deaf or hard of hearing child needs this book and so does every speech pathologist, audiologist, educator, and pediatrician. Families often find themselves thrown into what Fertman calls 'some truly hellacious bureaucracy,' with a kid who urgently needs them to make high stakes choices. Too often they either get very little guidance or, worse, terrible advice and pseudoscience from misguided professionals. Fertman's book offers families an easy-to-read guide that cuts through the chaos, giving families essential, evidence-based tools they need to help their children thrive. They say babies don't come with an instruction manual, but now deaf and hard of hearing babies do."
—**Dr. Naomi Caselli**, assistant professor of Deaf Education and co-director, The Deaf Center at Boston University

"I love the matter-of-fact way *The Deaf Baby Instruction Manual* shares information. More families need access to information about the IEP and IFSP processes in the way Will Fertman presents them!"
—**Caitlin Stueve**, DHHS-P, speech-language pathologist and board member, California Hands and Voices

"Fertman's candid, no-nonsense style is well complemented by his sensitivity to the confusion and concern many parents experience when their child is identified as deaf or hard of hearing. The quick start guide at the beginning is a clear and concise rundown of the most important points parents need to know while they're still reeling and sleep deprived, and his recommendations for how to sign with a baby are right on! He explains clearly how to capture and hold a baby's attention and take advantage of ASL's rich visual expression to get language going and to bond with your child through the process of learning ASL."
—**Dr. Razi M. Zarchy**, professor of communication sciences and disorders, California State University, Sacramento

"If you have been around the block in Deaf mainstream educational settings, or ever confronted the audism or misguided good intentions there, you will be stunned by this book. It is funny, totally irreverent, compassionate, and direct. Will Fertman is a great writer and an amazing father, but the power in this book lies in the shock of seeing someone telling the truth, strongly and unequivocally, and prioritizing absolutely nothing but the wellbeing of Deaf children. . . . Compassion is part of the book's power. Fertman truly understands and supports parents' dilemmas and feelings, and they will sense that and respond by trusting—and listening—to him."

—**Rachel Zemach**, Deaf educator and author of *The Butterfly Cage*

The Deaf Baby Instruction Manual

A Guide for Parents of Deaf and Hard of Hearing Children from Birth Through Kindergarten

Will Fertman

BLOOMSBURY ACADEMIC
NEW YORK • LONDON • OXFORD • NEW DELHI • SYDNEY

BLOOMSBURY ACADEMIC
Bloomsbury Publishing Inc, 1359 Broadway, New York, NY 10018, USA
Bloomsbury Publishing Plc, 50 Bedford Square, London, WC1B 3DP, UK
Bloomsbury Publishing Ireland, 29 Earlsfort Terrace, Dublin 2, D02 AY28, Ireland

BLOOMSBURY, BLOOMSBURY ACADEMIC and the Diana logo are trademarks of
Bloomsbury Publishing Plc

First published in the United States of America 2026

Copyright © Will Fertman, 2026
Cover images: © istock/Mladen Zivkovic, © istock/millann, © istock/LumiNola, © istock/PeopleImages

All rights reserved. No part of this publication may be: i) reproduced or transmitted in any form, electronic or mechanical, including photocopying, recording or by means of any information storage or retrieval system without prior permission in writing from the publishers; or ii) used or reproduced in any way for the training, development or operation of artificial intelligence (AI) technologies, including generative AI technologies. The rights holders expressly reserve this publication from the text and data mining exception as per Article 4(3) of the Digital Single Market Directive (EU) 2019/790.

Bloomsbury Publishing Inc does not have any control over, or responsibility for, any third-party websites referred to or in this book. All internet addresses given in this book were correct at the time of going to press. The author and publisher regret any inconvenience caused if addresses have changed or sites have ceased to exist, but can accept no responsibility for any such changes.

A catalog record for this book is available from the Library of Congress.

ISBN: PB: 979-8-7651-8937-5
ePDF: 979-8-7651-8939-9
eBook: 979-8-7651-8938-2

Typeset by Deanta Global Publishing Services, Chennai, India
Printed and bound in the United States of America

For product safety related questions contact productsafety@bloomsbury.com.

To find out more about our authors and books visit www.bloomsbury.com and sign up for our newsletters.

*This book is dedicated to my family.
To Leo, who taught me how to be a father,
to Oscar, who taught me how to be the father of a deaf child,
to Minda, who learned parenthood alongside me,
and to Carrie and Rachel, who became family, too.
It is also dedicated my mother and father,
who raised me and my brother with so much love and care.*

Contents

Acknowledgments xi
Foreword xii
A Note on the Text xvi

Introduction: Congratulations, It's a Deaf Baby 1
    Now Skip to the Good Part 1
    Who Am I? 2
    Who Is This Book For? 2
    Ummm . . . Controversy? 3
    An Apology 4

1 Deaf Baby Quick Start Guide 7
    You're Going to Be Fine 7
    Frequently Asked Questions 10
    What Should I Do Next? 25

2 Day to Day with Your Deaf Baby 29
    How to Sign with a Baby 30
    Getting Attention 37
    Danger Alert! AKA, Sign Names 39
    Baby Care Basics 42
    Shopping 47
    Your Accessible Home 49
    Going Out 50
    Strollers, Carriers, and Car Seats 50
    Playgrounds 53

Playgroups, Finding, and Making 55
Errands 57
The Beach and the Pool 58
The Wilderness 62
Snow and Cold 64
Museums, Concerts, and Events 66
Reading to Your Deaf Child 67
ASL Children's Books and Media 74

3 Family 79
Dinner Table Syndrome: Not as Delicious as it Sounds 79
Siblings 86
Parents and Partners 94
Extended Family 98
Testers and Doubters 103
Cutting Ties 104
Family Heritage (Matzah Balls, etc.) 108
Home Culture / Deaf Culture 114
Religion 115

4 Doctors, Teachers, and Assholes 121
Deaf Ed Is Not a Guy 122
A Long and Boring History of Deaf Education in the United States 123
What's the Deal with Natural Languages, and What's the Problem with Sign Systems? 140
What's the Deal with Augmentative and Alternative Communication (AAC)? 148
Early Intervention, Special Education, and IDEA 149
IEP, IFSP, 504, WTF? 150
IFSP and IEP Quick Start Guide 152
IFSPs in Yet More Excruciating Detail 160
Assessments, Services, and Goals for IFSPs and IEPs 165
504 Plans: If You Really Loved Me, You Wouldn't Hurt Me 172
Dealing with Bad Professionals 174

Schools, Preschools, Daycares, and Sitters 184
Evaluating DHH Programs and Schools 190
Deaf Educational Philosophies 194
Mainstreaming 200
Educational Interpreters under IFSP, IEP, and 504 Plans 207
School Placement, FAPE, and the Problem with LRE 208
Tough Love versus Enough Love—Avoiding the Moonshot Mentality 210
Interpreters: Hiring and Firing 211
Medical Issues 217
Audiograms and the "Hearing Loss" Diagnosis 217
Health Concerns and Medical Testing 219
Hearing Devices Quick Start Guide 227
Cochlear Implant FAQ 232
CIs Now and Later 238
Hearing Aid, CROS, and BAHA FAQ 240
Fucking Magnets, How Do They Work? 243
How the Hell Am I Going to Pay for All This? 244

5 Dealing with It 247
Anger 247
Last Story Before Bed 251

Glossary 253
Social Terms 253
Medical and Audiological Terms 256
A Field Guide to Professionals 260
Index 265
About the Author 271

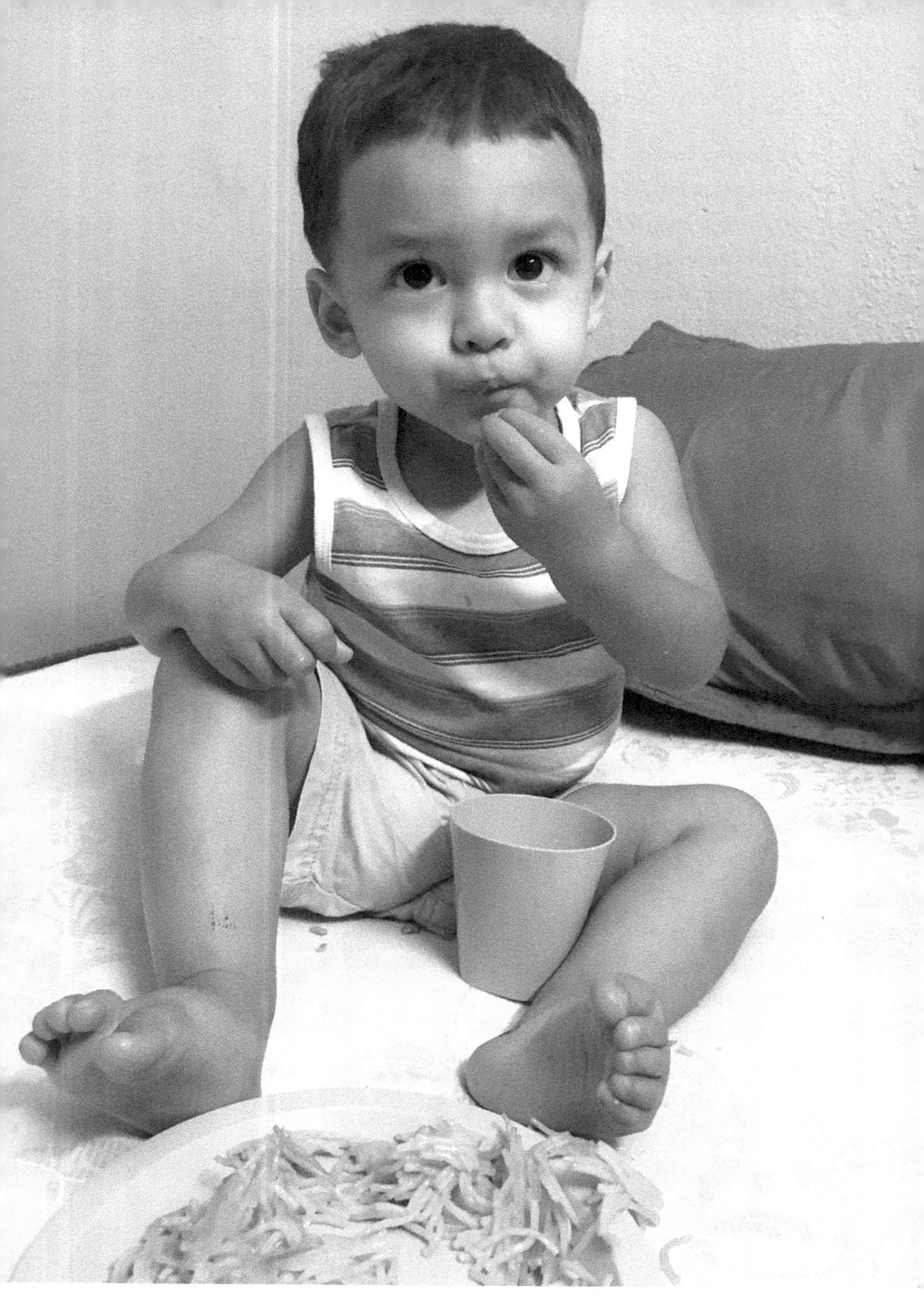

Stephanie Lucero, 2025

Acknowledgments

This book would not have been possible without the advice, support, education and example of many professionals, parents and humans, Deaf and hearing.

Rachel Zemach	Bee Vicars	Tracey
Susan Gonzalez	Leah Geer	Torrie
Kelly McCrary	Razi Zarchy	Kris
Malage LeBlanc	Caitlin Stueve	Joy
Christina Litzau	Sara Kennedy	Jay
Michele Berke	Emily Saltarelli	Molly
Julie Rems-Smario	Sarah Power	Johanna
Laura T. Petersen	Lauren Lamoureux	Tenysa
Rhys McGovern	Mark Drolsbaugh	Noel
Iva Ikeda	Sara Nović	Rachel
Gerardo Di Pietro	Aure Schrock	Jennifer
Wyatte Hall	Jen Nadol	John
Naomi Caselli	Lawrence Siegel	Barrett
Leala Holcomb	Carrie	Sara
Paddy Ladd	Lisa	Sam
Don Grushkin	Marisa	The staff, parents, and
Kim Ofori-Sanzo	Alina	students of CSD Fremont
Mallorie Evans	James	The staff of DCARA

Foreword

Dr. Kimberly Ofori-Sanzo

I met Will, as one does these days, online. Parents of deaf and hard of hearing children often seek advice on social media, and Will's responses to them were always kind, thoughtful, and evidence-based. We shared a passion for ensuring that these children acquire language and develop into their best selves, so I was honored when he asked me to write this foreword.

My journey started with a master's degree in speech-language pathology (SLP) from Gallaudet, the world's preeminent Deaf university. After graduating, I worked at a school for the deaf for nine years, where I witnessed firsthand the miseducation that medical and educational professionals provide to parents. Time and again, the use of fearmongering and the illusion of choice pushed parents into making decisions that were not in the best interests of their children.

Hearing parents were often explicitly told not to learn or use a signed language—a decision that can significantly impact their child's linguistic, cognitive, and socioemotional skills. Incomplete access to a first language at birth is known as language deprivation, and it has serious and lifelong repercussions for children's development. This was exacerbated by issues such as language neglect ("dinner table syndrome"), when a deaf or hard-of-hearing child is excluded from conversations in their direct environment. All of this had a cumulative effect on their health and well-being.

My experience as an SLP showed me the undeniable harm language deprivation and language neglect were having on my students, corroborating a growing body of scientific literature. To better help them, I went on to earn my doctorate in speech-language pathology and founded Language First, an organization that provides parents and professionals with research-backed information about raising deaf and hard-of-hearing children and supporting their language acquisition.

For a long time, I wished there was some sort of manual we could hand to parents to help them navigate this journey, which is so rife with misinformation and fear. Now, there is! Will's book is funny and relatable and will doubtless help ease some of the worries hearing parents have about their deaf child. However, most importantly, it is *accurate*. Will has the unique ability to explain concepts in a way that is comprehensible and digestible. The information in this guide is not only on the mark, but vitally important for hearing parents to know. It is a must-read for anyone who has just been told that their child has any degree of reduced hearing.

Dr. Kimberly Ofori-Sanzo is co-founder of the American Board of Deaf and Hard of Hearing Specialists and the founder of Language First, an organization that advocates for ASL/English bilingualism and the importance of a strong first language foundation for deaf and hard of hearing children.

Dr. Wyatte Hall

> I am Deaf. My family does not sign. This has defined our relationship my whole life.
>
> I only have superficial conversations with my parents:
>
> "How's work?"
>
> "Good."

I see in their faces the desire to know more and their pain when I can't give it to them. The pain is preferable to the extreme awkwardness of trying to have a real conversation. My sister and I do not talk—despite my repeated requests over the years for her to learn sign, she never has. Until her death several years ago, my grandmother would whisper something into my ear every time she left a family event. To this day, I have no idea what she said to me; I imagine it was something sweet and loving, but it literally fell on deaf ears.

Because of this dynamic, I was often the last to know anything in my family. My sister would get the facts first; my mom would sometimes relay them to me later out of guilt. So, in fact, I did not know a lot about my parents' experience having me until I was an adult—my hearing wife actually learned the details before I did.

I was born in Washington, D.C. in 1986. My parents learned that I was deaf in 1988, the year of the Deaf President Now protests at Gallaudet University, which was just down the street from our home. Despite the wealth of Deaf expertise and knowledge on their doorstep, my parents chose to put me in a D.C. special education program with just hearing aids.

We moved to the Albany, NY, area when I was five. I arrived in kindergarten testing at the level of a three-and-a-half-year-old and was placed in a mainstream total communication program. The story is that I caught up in six months and remained at grade level ever since. While the total communication approach was not an immersive American Sign Language environment and devoid of Deaf role models, I believe the *signing* and visual access to communication saved me. Even with that, I did not fully find myself as a whole person until I started going to Deaf summer camps and then to college where ASL was available.

Please understand, my parents did a lot for me. They advocated fiercely for my education and they did not accept low expectations. They gave me everything I needed as a child, except the one thing I needed the most.

Among the many half-lies you might hear as a parent, one of the most common is that if you allow your deaf child to sign, you will lose them to the Deaf community. The opposite is true. Of my peers, the ones who have the best relationships with their parents and siblings are those who had a family that allowed them to fully embrace who they are as a whole deaf person, meeting them where they are by signing with them and giving them full access to Deaf friends and adults. Every time I see that, I can't help but look on with jealousy and, frankly, some resentment. That's the resentment that becomes a wedge between families and their adult deaf children, giving a hint of truth to the myth that a signing child will abandon their hearing family.

Give your deaf child everything, including the language of signs. They will return the investment to you a thousandfold.

Dr. Wyatte Hall is Assistant Professor of Public Health Sciences, Pediatrics, Obstetrics & Gynecology, Neurology, and Center for Community Health and Prevention at the University of Rochester Medical Center. He directs the Visual Language Access and Acquisition Lab as a leading researcher on the relationship between childhood language experiences and quality of life outcomes in deaf children and adults. In 2025, he was named to Forbes' inaugural Accessibility 100 list, recognizeing top innovators and impact-makers in the field of accessibility.

A Note on the Text

In this book, I'm using the word "deaf" as a catch-all. There's a wide range of hearing levels among kids, and a lot of vocabulary describing various medical and social flavors of deafness—*deaf, Deaf, hearing loss, hard of hearing, D/HH, Deaf Disabled, microtia and atresia, unilateral deafness, DeafBlind, CHARGE syndrome, auditory neuropathy, bilateral sensorineural reverse cookie bite hearing loss*, and so on. However, there are also similarities in the experiences these kids and their families have. In general, when I write little-d "deaf," I mean children and adults who don't have typical hearing, whatever the reason, hearing level, or language they use. When I write big-D "Deaf," I'm talking about deaf people who embrace Deaf culture and sign language (generally ASL in this book).

Also note that the terms "hearing impaired" and "hearing loss" are considered to be offensive by many Deaf adults, but "hearing loss" is still used widely by doctors and in a lot of official documentation. I use it in my book only when referring to a medical diagnosis or to a situation where someone's hearing levels are declining—"progressive hearing loss." There's more about this in the glossary at the back.

Finally, whenever you see whole words written in capital letters in this book, I'm referring to specific signs or words in American Sign Language—this is known as gloss. So if I write DUCK, I'm probably referring to the specific ASL sign for the bird; you don't have to get under the table. I don't especially like gloss because it makes ASL seem shouty and pissed off, when in reality, it can be incredibly tender and sweet—I put my kid to bed with ASL, after all. It's the standard though, and I'm not the guy to change it.

Introduction
Congratulations, It's a Deaf Baby

If you're a hearing parent or caregiver who's discovered your child is deaf or hard of hearing, let me be the first to say congratulations! Everything's going to be OK, and please send pictures—they are so cute.

You might have already started getting information handed to you about your kid. It can seem overwhelming, but honestly, there are only three things to know about deaf infants and children:

1. All kids need to learn at least one language by about age three.
2. Deaf and hard of hearing kids don't have typical hearing, so learning spoken languages can be a lot harder for them.
3. Learning sign language is a lot easier for them, so start there.

That's it.

There's other stuff in the book about hearing technology, school and family dynamics, some fussy details about flicking the lights, and one surprise historical supervillain waiting in the wings. But it all pretty much flows from those three principles.

Now Skip to the Good Part

I've set up the book to be accessible to time-pressed, middle-of-the-night-feeding, worried-to-death parents. **If you have no other time, just go to Part**

1 and read the *Quick Start Guide*. These are the basics. The other chapters are for when you're getting some rest.

There are additional quick start guides later in the book for urgent-but-boring topics like IEPs, cochlear implants, and more, but just get through that first chapter for now. You're going to be fine, and you will have *fun*.

Who Am I?

My name is Will, I'm the hearing father of two boys, one hearing and one deaf. I live with them and my beautiful wife in Northern California.

Having a deaf baby was a major surprise to my family, and we struggled to find any truly basic guides for hearing parents. We did scare the shit out of ourselves reading some outdated books from the 1970s and watching *A Quiet Place* (protip: *don't do it*). But what worked best for us was seeking out advice from the experts: Deaf adults, and particularly Deaf scientists, language, and education professionals. This book is a synthesis of their advice, backed up with current research on best practices, along with my family's personal experience. If you have questions about anything you read in this book, or want more information, you can contact me at willfertman.com—but please just ask a Deaf adult. They know better than I do.

Who Is This Book For?

This book is for hearing parents or caregivers of babies and young children aged five and under, who've been identified as deaf or hard of hearing, or are getting their hearing tested now, **or who are worried that their kid is deaf but haven't been able to confirm it.**

On that last point: these days, all infants born in US hospitals should get a newborn hearing screening. That's great when it works, but even if everything is done properly, deaf kids frequently slip through. Like all medical tests, newborn screens aren't 100 percent accurate, and even if they were, it's very common for babies to be born with progressive hearing loss; what's a hearing baby at one week can be a deaf baby at six months, and it can be fiendishly difficult to tell what an infant can and can't hear in general. They can keep you guessing for *years*.

Because of this, and because of the glacial pace of insurance approvals and audiological testing, parents will often know something isn't right a long time before they get medical confirmation. If you think your child is deaf or hard of hearing, or you're stuck in limbo between medical appointments, **you don't have to wait to see the next doctor, speech pathologist, audiologist, educator, or social worker to start helping your baby**. You can do a huge amount to help them develop language and cognitive skills right now by learning sign language and using it with them.

This book is for your hard of hearing child. Some hearing professionals will make a big distinction between groups of kids who are "really deaf" and those who are hard of hearing, or who "only have some hearing loss." This isn't actually a thing—there's no bright line where a hard of hearing kid becomes officially deaf. It's a matter of personal preference how someone identifies, but deaf and hard of hearing children draw from the same toolbox of strategies to get by in the world, and parents of deaf and hard of hearing kids need to know the same facts.

There are also kids with typical hearing who benefit from using sign language and deaf educational approaches—some children on the autism spectrum, kids with receptive or expressive language disorders, and more. If that describes your child, I hope this book can be of help to you, too.

Ummm . . . Controversy?

You may have heard that there's a little disagreement about raising and educating deaf kids. Much of this comes from conflict between advocates of spoken language and advocates of sign language. You'll see pretty quickly where I fall on the big debate, but let me be totally clear: our goal here isn't "your child must speak" or "your child must sign." The goal is to raise an independent, self-confident adult who can do their own laundry and date people you don't approve of. Go to school, get a career, find a partner, and give you adorable grandchildren (or not—no pressure).

This means giving your child strong language skills, good academic options, and friends, peers, and mentors that they can turn to for support. Because even when you've forbidden it, they will still need *someone* holding their hand when they get that SpongeBob tattoo on their ass. This applies whether they end up using sign language, spoken language, hearing aids, cochlear implants, or all of the above in their daily life.

An Apology

I want to issue an apology ahead of time to parents whose deaf children have additional disabilities. About 30 percent of deaf kids have them, and they are a very diverse group with an array of needs. Since I don't have experience or expertise in the area, and because there are so many different considerations to add on, I can only give some superficial advice, and I'm sure to miss things. If this book survives into a second edition, I hope to add more perspectives from the Deaf + and Deaf Disabled community.

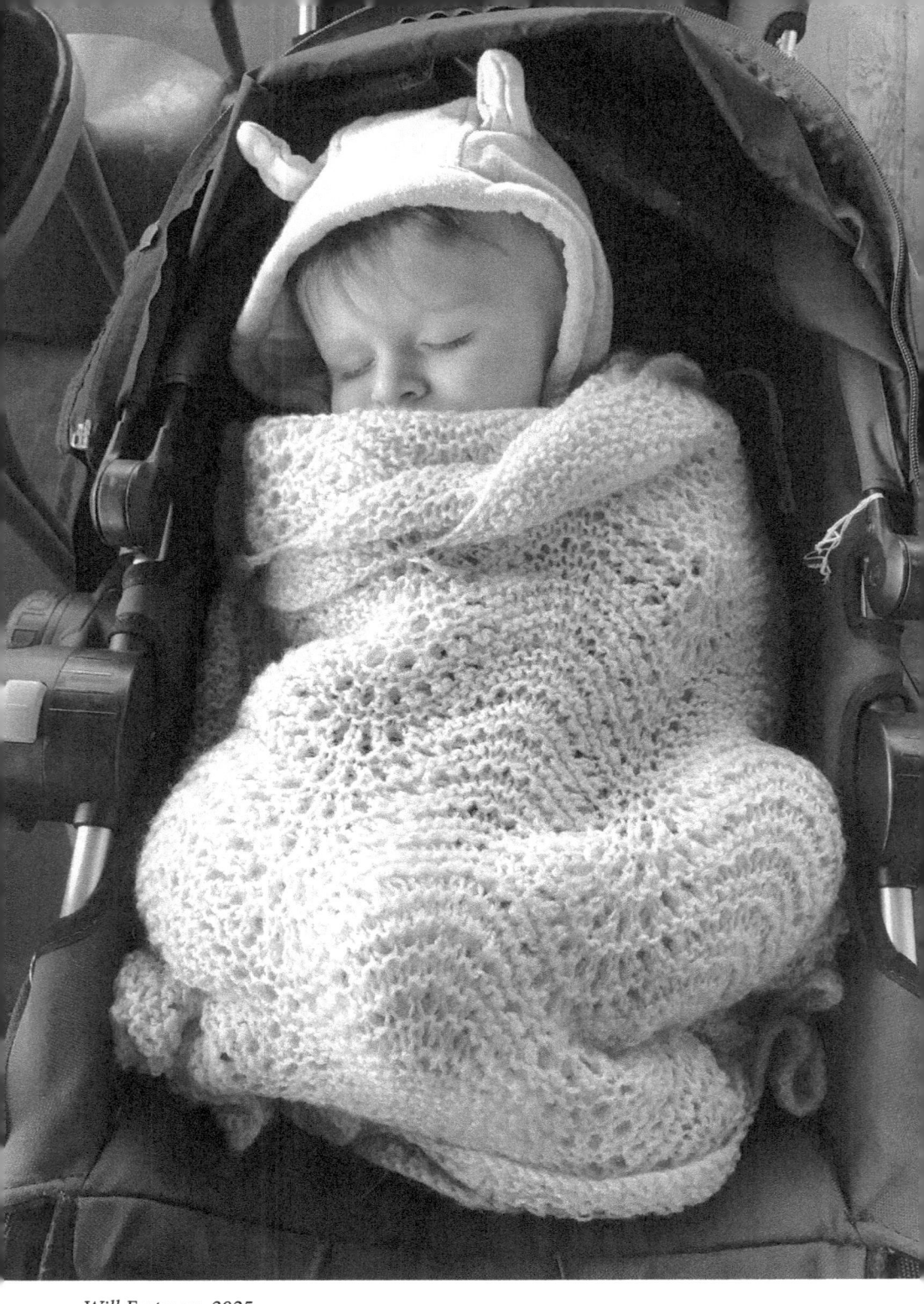

Will Fertman, 2025

1

Deaf Baby Quick Start Guide

Potty training my two-year-old.

He poops, looks into the potty, looks back at me wide-eyed.

He signs MOUNTAIN.

I'm so proud.

You're Going to Be Fine

Only about 1 in 500 newborns is identified as deaf or hard of hearing, but 90 percent of those deaf babies are born to hearing parents. No wonder you were surprised.

Because childhood deafness is so rare, doctors and audiologists don't always do a great job explaining the situation to hearing parents. This is a shame, because the situation is actually pretty good. In case you didn't read the introduction (who does?), there are only three essential things you need to know:

All Children Need to Learn *at Least* One Language by About Age Three

All children, hearing and deaf, are hard-wired to acquire languages. In fact, babies need exposure to a natural language for their brains to develop properly.

The time between birth and about three years old is a critical period when a baby must learn that first language, usually abbreviated as their *L1*.

A child's L1 gives them a toolkit to use when they're trying to organize their own thoughts, guess what other people are thinking, and learn new things. Learning a language is essential for their cognitive growth—it cannot be skipped or delayed without harming them. But given a strong first language, typically developing deaf kids will be equal to their hearing peers in every way except, you know, the hearing.

On the other hand, kids who miss the 0–3 language window and don't acquire an L1 until they're older can experience reasoning and learning deficits that persist into adulthood. This is known as *language deprivation syndrome*. Language deprivation causes difficulties not just with learning an L1 later, but also with math, logic, and social skills. It's a form of neurological damage, much easier to prevent than it is to treat, and it's the first major issue you want to avoid with your deaf child.

If you're reading this and your older-than-three child is language delayed or has recently been identified as deaf, please know that although language deprivation is serious, it can be helped by professionals specifically trained in the treatment of deaf children with language deprivation—but *not* just a random speech-language pathologist or teacher of the deaf! Getting accessible language started as soon as you can will definitely help, but language deprivation may be an ongoing obstacle for your child, and it's something we're trying to avoid whenever possible.

Deaf Kids Can't Hear, So Learning Spoken Languages Can Be a Lot Harder for Them

No kidding, right?

If you've got typical hearing, you probably picked up your first language from your parents, family, and caregivers, starting at birth. You didn't take a class; you learned by playing and imitating. You listened to the people around you and to your own voice as you babbled. Bit by bit, you built up a *receptive* vocabulary—understanding words. At the same time, you were copying the sounds other people made and began to string it all together into an *expressive* vocabulary—saying words. Your baby brain absorbed language like your baby body absorbed milk: more or less effortlessly.

A deaf infant does not have easy access to spoken language for picking up that L1. Even if your child is only hard of hearing, words that others say might come through too garbled to tell one from another, and your child may not be able to clearly hear the sounds that they make themselves. There isn't a seamless feedback loop of sound, voice, and meaning.

It can be tricky to imagine the situation from your baby's perspective—after all, if you're reading this, you already *have* language. A deaf infant's challenge goes beyond just not hearing words, it's not having a foundation of meaning to build on. Whatever strategies you or I might use to fill in a missed syllable or piece of information aren't available to them. So, for a deaf kid, acquiring a first language through residual hearing or lip-reading is work; potentially a lot of work, and often impossible, even when helped by technology.

Learning Sign Language Is a Lot Easier for Deaf Kids, So Start There

Natural signed languages like American Sign Language (ASL) are visual languages, entirely taken up by the eyes. A baby with typical vision will pick up a sign language just as easily as a spoken language, by watching parents and caregivers sign to them and to each other. They will then naturally start babbling with their fingers (which is *adorable*), and play with words, copy adults, express their needs, pick up nursery rhymes, and generally do all the baby language stuff. Once they have that effortless access, the language-learning feedback loop can happen.

And once a child has begun to build those deep cognitive skills in their L1, they can naturally transfer those skills to other languages (L2, L3, etc.). You might encounter misguided professionals who insist that you should only stick to spoken English, but research shows that learning ASL will actually help your child learn English or any other language that you teach them.

Frequently Asked Questions

Where Do I Start?

Go hug your baby. Deaf infants need everything hearing infants need: lots of milk, lots of cuddles, regular burping, peek-a-boo sessions, hats with animal ears,[1] the whole nine yards.. Take a minute to smell their head and admire their tiny face. Kids need love most of all, and you already know how to love them; it's the basic communication that everything else is built on.

The difference with deaf kids is that you'll need to add new layers of communication, learning them alongside your baby. But don't worry, it's not a mysterious process. Every child, deaf or hearing, gives us new things to learn. It's just that with deaf kids, the lessons come from unexpected places.

Sign Language, What's the Deal?

You probably already know the basics: signed languages are languages that use the hands, face, and body to express words and sentences, rather than the voice. Different countries and communities use different sign languages, but they all do one thing—swap vision and movement for hearing and speech as the *modality* of the language.

Natural sign languages are full languages in and of themselves—they're not just miming or gesturing. They have their own vocabulary, syntax, and grammar, and aren't a word-for-word translation of a spoken language "on the hands." In American Sign Language, for instance, the word order can be different from English, but different is fine: sign languages work perfectly as an L1 for kids, deaf *or* hearing. In fact, learning one is a powerful first step your deaf child will make toward mastering English.

What Sign Language Should I Learn?

If you're reading this in the United States or Anglophone Canada, learn American Sign Language (ASL). It's the most common language used by the

---

[1] Or hats that look like vegetables; your choice.

Deaf community here.[2] But just like spoken languages, sign languages differ from country to country, and countries with the same spoken language can actually have *different* sign languages. ASL, for instance, has more in common with the sign languages of France (LSF) and Mexico (LSM) than it does with British (BSL) or Australian sign (Auslan).

What's Up with "Natural" Sign Languages?

A natural language is one that grew unplanned in a community of people, passed on between the generations. Whether they're spoken or signed, all natural languages share a very high level of sophistication—they're an expression of the human brain's deep neurological development. So even though ASL is different from English, Yiddish, Arabic, Japanese, Irish Sign Language, or Kenyan Sign Language, each of these languages can communicate complex ideas and feelings, describe events and objects, and get their point across equally well.

ASL itself has been spoken in the United States for more than two hundred years, passed down between generations of Deaf users. It's full of the things you'd find in any language: dirty jokes, grammar snobs, poetry, talk shows, regional accents, and about a million synonyms for the word "pizza."

What About . . .

...Signed Exact English (SEE)?
...Manually Coded English (MCE)?
...Pidgin Signed English (PSE)?
...Makaton?
...Sign Supported English (SSE)?
...Cued English / Cued Speech, etc.?

In the deaf education world, you will run into plenty of artificial sign systems that were invented, like Klingon or Elvish, and didn't develop naturally within

---

[2]Not the *only* one, though. There are many other sign languages native to North America, including indigenous sign languages like Plains Sign Language and Inuit Sign Language, Black American Sign Language, *Lengua de señas mexicana*, *Langue des signes du Québec*, and many more—the world is cool.

a community. These were mostly created to help deaf kids learn to speak or write English, or as limited communication tools for special purposes.

Sign systems are not natural languages and aren't a good choice for your kid's L1. Although they are mostly based on English and seem language-like, they actually lack elements your child needs to develop a strong cognitive foundation for learning. Like food without vitamins, they can deprive your child's brain of crucial nutrients needed to grow. Some kids do ok with some of these systems or use them for specific things, but when taught as a first language, they put your child at higher risk for language problems, including language deprivation.

Sign systems are not common outside of educational settings, and you won't find a large community of Deaf adults or interpreters using them. Because of this, learning one as an L1 can not only set kids back developmentally but also be socially isolating to boot.

I'll give overviews of all these in a later chapter, but for now, just know that if you encounter hearing teachers or professionals pushing a sign system for your child's L1, this is a big red flag—avoid these programs and professionals if you can.

What about Baby Sign?

Baby sign is a frustrating thing. I'm not talking about ASL courses, books, or resources for parents of deaf children, created by Deaf instructors. Those are awesome. What I'm talking about are the baby-and-parent lessons—original Baby Signs® brand or not—that you see promoted for *hearing* children in books, websites, and social media by hearing teachers.

The baby sign trend started taking off in the early 2000s, and the idea is simple and basically correct: hearing babies can learn to use signs before they learn to talk, and this can help reduce frustration in pre-verbal kids and support spoken language growth. We actually used baby sign with our first son, who is hearing, and it worked like a charm: Leo knew EAT, MORE, ALL DONE, and a bunch of other words long before he could speak, and it was easy for him to express himself and get what he needed.

So far, so good. But this kind of baby sign has problems—big problems:

The words taught in baby sign classes might not be real ASL, or any other sign language. Hearing folks who teach baby sign often have only a shallow understanding of natural sign languages, so they make up or modify whatever signs they want in any way that they want. For a parent of a deaf child, it means that you're teaching your child gibberish . . . or worse.

Baby sign has ya'll out here signing BLOWJOB for "oatmeal." Learn ASL from Deaf folks and stop spreading that nonsense, please.

Lisa Cryer, Deaf educational advocate

They don't teach grammar or other language structures. Signs are almost always meant to be dropped in one at a time as visual support to spoken sentences and songs. It's fine for hearing children who are getting plenty of language exposure anyway, but it doesn't give a deaf baby access to full language, just a small jumble of disconnected words.

It's a giant *screw you* to the Deaf community. Taking their cherished language, one often denied to deaf children, chopping it up, sprinkling it with fake words, and selling it back to unsuspecting hearing parents is really low.

If you're like me, you might already know some baby sign from a previous kid or other childcare experience. If so, you might have to relearn some things. Better not to be like me in the first place: find a real ASL class, and don't do baby sign.

Ok, You Sold Me on ASL. Can I Teach My Kid English Too?

Yes! You can, and you should. English literacy is massively important for your kid's future, and there is no reason a deaf child can't develop age-appropriate English skills and be strong readers and writers if they have ASL as a solid L1. If your child has access through their hearing devices, they can learn spoken English *at the same time* they learn ASL—that whole L1, L2 numbering system is a little misleading.

And if your family *doesn't* use English at home, you can teach them your home language, too! Heritage languages are important connections with family culture, and kids can actually learn tons of languages at once. In many parts of the world, they grow up with two or three in the home before they even arrive at school.

Be warned again: some professionals will tell you that teaching sign language will interfere with learning a spoken language. That's completely backwards: **studies have repeatedly shown that deaf kids—even kids with hearing aids and CIs—who get early exposure to ASL are more likely to have age-appropriate English skills, comparable to their hearing peers.**

Whether your kid can develop strong *speech* skills is another matter . . .

Will My Kid Talk? Will They Have a "Deaf Accent?"

Maybe. For deaf children, acquiring speech, let alone "clear" speech, can range from straightforward to impossible. It depends on a lot of factors—residual hearing levels, technology, their anatomy, how much your kid actually enjoys it, and more. Like any talent, some kids have the knack, but for others, learning to speak can be like learning to write with invisible ink—frustrating and pointless.

It's important to remember that language is what goes on in your brain, not what comes out of your mouth. For your child to develop a strong cognitive-linguistic foundation, speech isn't actually key; they need a language that's as easy as breathing to play with and build up those deep neurological structures. Ultimately, language is how they will understand themselves, other people, and the world. Speech without language is just blowing air.

Many Deaf adults have painful memories of putting in long hours in speech therapy or at oral schools, working on spoken English to the exclusion of everything else—math, history, social studies, art, flirting—just to end up with a skill that only takes them halfway to communicating with the hearing world, if that:

> Speech therapists can sometimes mislead parents and youth about their progress. Many young adults leave programs thinking their speech skills are clear and intelligible only to encounter communication barriers in the world outside therapy offices.
>
> They often find through those barriers that a limited number of people will understand them simply because of the familiarity between them. That familiarity does not exist with the world at large.
>
> Susan Gonzalez, Deaf educational advocate

Speech can be a very emotional issue because people are often judged by their voices. Folks with strong accents or difficult-to-understand pronunciation can be seen as less smart and less capable. No matter what choices we make about speech for our kids, none of us wants them to be looked down on, and we all want them to have the chance to socialize with peers and navigate the hearing world around them. Strong speaking skills can sometimes help in that regard—but not always:

> Hearing people assume that having "good speech" is a good thing, and that the less Deaf-accented one's voice sounds, the better. But if I start talking with someone with my "good speech," they will talk back, even if I am telling them it won't work.
>
> Let's say I encounter my neighbor, and say "Hello."
>
> "*Wegga nee ackaby!*" The woman replies.
>
> "Look, I am Deaf. I can't understand you," I say, pleasantly.
>
> I often offer alternative methods. But because I can speak, in her heart of hearts, the dots simply don't connect for her, and she believes I can also hear.
>
> "*Will I coodocumena da hip,*" she replies, and, despite my blank and questioning face, she continues.
>
> Rachel Zemach, Deaf author and educator

If you want to pursue speech for your kid, it's a "would be nice" goal, rather than a must-have. You will want to start early and find a speech-language pathologist (SLP) who's fun, who doesn't discourage ASL, and who won't turn you and your kid's life into a 24/7 therapy session. If your child hates it, or if it's taking up more than an hour or two a week, dip out—see my chapter on *Dealing with Bad Professionals* for more on recognizing and managing bad SLPs.

Will My Kid Learn to Read Lips?

Maybe. Lip-reading is a dicey thing, and movies and TV exaggerate how well it works. Only about thirty percent of the English language is visible on a speaker's lips, and it takes a lot of guesswork and residual hearing to fill in the rest—an overall process more properly called *speechreading*. Mustaches are a problem. Strangers, mumblers, head-turners, soft-talkers, over-annunciators all make things harder, too. Some deaf people rely on it for their day-to-day interactions, but many find it exhausting or just too difficult, and even skillful speechreaders can prefer to use other ways of communicating. So it's a cool skill if you're a spy, and it may be something your child will use in the future, especially in conjunction with hearing technology, but it is not the way to get your child their first language.

Note that some oral deaf programs and speech-language pathologists make speechreading a major component of their teaching, but many have moved on to the even more painful and pointless Auditory-Verbal Therapy (AVT), which actually forbids speechreading and relies entirely on using sound from hearing aids or CIs. Although AVT is taught in professional training programs, research shows that it's not any more effective than run-of-the-mill speech-language therapy. And because it typically discourages or forbids learning sign language, AVT can put your child at greater jeopardy of language deprivation. Just like sign systems, be extremely wary of anyone pushing AVT or its parent philosophy, Listening and Spoken Language (LSL).

What If I'm Not Good at Sign Language (AKA, What If I Sucked at French in High School?)

Welcome to the club. I've been studying ASL for years and I'm still tripping over my thumbs. Here's a secret, though: **you don't have to be instantly fluent in ASL to support your kid's ASL development.**

Studies demonstrate that hearing parents who start learning ASL early on with their deaf children end up with kids who have strong overall language skills, comparable to typical hearing babies. Learning alongside your kid is key. Recent estimates say that hearing parents who have the skills of a first- to second-year ASL student by the time their child is eighteen months, and of a third- to fourth-year ASL student by the time their kid is five, have children with fully age-appropriate language. You can swing that.

Learning will take time: the rule of thumb is that it takes at least seven years to become really comfortable in a new language, but honestly, just in terms of communicating with your baby, you can learn the signs for MOM, DAD, MILK, DIAPER, and I LOVE YOU in about thirty seconds. You don't have to become a handtalk ninja overnight, you just have to keep at it.

What about Hearing Aids or Cochlear Implants?

Right now, there are a number of different tools out there that might give a deaf kid more access to sound. Depending on your child's situation, hearing aids (HAs), bone-anchored hearing aids (BAHAs), or cochlear implants (CIs) might be recommended by your doctor, audiologist, or a nosy stranger on the bus.[3]

It's important to know that every kid is different. Some technology doesn't work for some forms of deafness, or not well enough to give children access to spoken language, and some kids just won't like using their hearing devices. Even babies with identical diagnoses don't react the same way to a given device.

While modern hearing technology is remarkable, don't let the professionals fool you: many of the factors that determine how well it works are outside of your—and your audiologist's—control. My son has cochlear implants that he likes, and they have allowed him a lot of access to spoken English. He has peers who got all the same services, devices, and opportunities who have gotten little or no benefit from them.

Here's the kicker, though: even if they work for your child in the sound booth, hearing prosthetics are not a reliable way to give your child their first language. Let me repeat that: **depending only on technology to give your kid access to their first language is a gamble, and losing that bet can be devastating to your child's developing brain.**

This is a problem because it is so hard to measure what a baby actually hears. The audiologist's tests can give you an idea of tones and frequencies, but there's a big difference between hearing a beep in a booth and being able

---

[3]There are also less common CROS and BiCROS systems, middle ear implants (MEI), auditory brainstem implants (ABI), and probably some other stuff that a nosy stranger knows about that I don't.

to follow fluent speech in the real world. On top of that, expressive speech—talking—lags receptive speech—understanding words—by months and years. Babies with typical hearing are receiving language from birth, but are not expected to express their first word until twelve months old or later. Deaf babies may not have their hearing device situation sorted out by then—*they may not even be identified as deaf yet*—but the language window is already one-third gone.

By the time we're able to get accurate measures of language acquisition, you're already playing catch-up. The timeline is just too short between identification of deafness and that year-three deadline. Given that the effects of language deprivation can be lifelong and debilitating, that's a bad bet. So whatever options are open for your child with technology, you also need to pursue sign language.

What about Gene Therapy?

Don't bet on that, either. As of this writing, there have been a couple of gene therapy studies out that were partially effective in reversing specific kinds of genetically linked deafness. While the technology is moving fast, it will be many years before these therapies are fully tested for safety and efficacy, and they may never be approved for your child's particular flavor. I discuss gene therapy more in Part 4, but the language window is brief, and waiting around is not an option.

What If . . .

. . . my kid is only hard of hearing, or has mild or moderate deafness?
. . . my kid is only deaf in one ear (aka single-sided deafness (SSD) or unilateral deafness)?
. . . my kid has progressive hearing loss, but can hear pretty well right now?
. . . hearing aids or cochlear implants work really well for them?

You should still learn ASL with them.

Every child has different needs, and there are folks with all kinds of deafness who manage in the hearing world without using sign language. But you can't guess ahead of time if your child will be one of these people, and what tools they might *want* to use. Frankly, the world is also full of deaf folks whose parents were assured that the hearing aid / CI / oral education / lip-reading scheme they were giving their child was going to be enough, and it wasn't.

One thing to know is that progressive hearing loss is common among hard of hearing children, and it's not always possible to predict when their hearing levels will drop again. Giving kids with mild or moderate deafness access to sign language early, when it's easiest for them to learn, is much better than waiting until they "really" need it.

Also keep in mind that kids who have mild or single-sided deafness can still have very noticeable gaps in their spoken language acquisition. Although the balance of their education may be tipped toward English, ASL can help plug those holes.

The truth is that many deaf people have some level of hearing, especially with modern hearing tech. But because deafness is often a question of loss of detail, not just volume, there's a huge difference between *hearing a lot of sound* and being able to easily understand speech. Again, it boils down to effort—you want to have an effortless language channel open to your child, even if it's an option they only use sometimes.

Imagine your kid can understand seventy-five percent of a spoken conversation:

A lot of %^$@! can get lost &%$# you cut 25 ^$#*@ of the words $%& of a normal *%$&^%$#. It's not impossible ^&% figure out the $!@ from context, but &!@#! it all day !*%^$, for your entire *^%$^% can be exhausting.

Now imagine your child understands only sixty percent of what's said. Or fifty. You can see how even mild deafness can shut kids out from opportunities to learn and socialize, and it can definitely disrupt the acquisition of an L1.

The real world isn't the audiologist's office. There are all kinds of situations where it's much harder to hear: on the playground, in a classroom, at a restaurant, and more. Your child's "very good" receptive skills in the testing booth may become "very crappy" when they're at Chuck E. Cheese. My own kid is a good example: he likes wearing his CIs, he talks a lot, and has strong receptive English skills. But at a noisy birthday party, or on a windy beach? Get those hands up, 'cause he's not gonna understand you.

What If My Kid Can't Use Their Hands to Sign?

If your deaf child has a motor disability or anatomical difference that affects their hands, they may not be able to fully employ expressive sign language. This is sometimes taken to mean that they shouldn't be exposed to sign language at all. The truth is, while they might need to use sign approximations, speech, or augmentative and alternative communication (AAC) like picture boards or computer programs to express themselves, if they are deaf, they still need a receptive language that's 100 percent accessible to them.

Kids who only have one hand to sign with are in a different situation. ASL is totally expressible one-handed, but your child will probably benefit from having role models who sign one-handed to see what their specific strategies are.

What If My Kid Is Also Blind or Low Vision?

There are several options available for children who are deafblind or otherwise don't have typical sight. For kids with a limited field of vision, ASL can be signed in such a way that your hands stay fully in view. For many children with low vision, this adapted ASL is their L1. For kids with very little visual access, ASL has also been adapted for touch—this is known as Tactile ASL or TASL, which uses hand-to-hand contact to translate visual signs into touch.

Then there is the very awesome ProTactile, which has been developed entirely by and for DeafBlind people in response to the limitations of TASLs visual-to-tactile approach. ProTactile has a separate vocabulary and grammar from ASL and uses more body contact to fully communicate ideas and emotions by touch. DeafBlind educator Jelica Nuccio and writer John Lee Clark are major advocates for ProTactile, and it's worth looking them up.

Deafblind children have a unique set of challenges, but the United States has a vibrant DeafBlind community. Find your state deafblind services agency and the National Center on Deafblindness, as well as the Protactile Language Interpreting National Education Program and deafblindkids.org for more information.

How Will *I* Learn Sign Language?

You can start learning ASL online right now—there's an index of resources up at willfertman.com—but in order to really progress, you're going to have to find a Deaf teacher, either in person or remotely. Live teachers can give critical feedback as you progress, and having a Deaf teacher gives you some confidence that you're learning the correct material; some hearing ASL "teachers" out there are, um, not good. It also shows respect for Deaf culture and introduces you to a Deaf adult who may have important insights for you as a hearing parent. You can find Deaf teachers in these convenient locations:

Early Intervention (EI) Services: In the United States, EI serves everyone with a deaf baby under the age of three. If you aren't already in touch, please look up your state's Early Intervention services now. You need them to get access to all the state services for your baby and family. There's a whole chapter on EI later in the book.

Some EI services will have Deaf mentors or ASL classes, or will be able to refer you to those services in a local school district or other locations. This is a good start, but you are just as likely to be dealing with a hearing teacher, and you are also likely to encounter either a program that has no sign language at all or offers an artificial sign system like SEE or Cued Speech that aren't natural languages. If that's the case, please find another source of ASL instruction for you and your kid.

At your local school for the deaf: State-supported deaf schools will often have ASL outreach classes for deaf kids, parents, and siblings, starting from birth onward. Not only can you learn the language, but you can also meet teachers and staff, parents, and playmates for your kids, and get a peek inside the school.

Deaf schools can offer a wide variety of classes and support groups for parents beyond just ASL, as well as events for the kids like playgroups or story times. You don't necessarily need to be enrolled or even in the same state—sometimes the closest school is over the border—so check 'em out!

At your local deaf services agency: There is a deaf services agency serving every community in the United States (although some cover huge territories), and they vary between state-run programs and independent nonprofits. These agencies will often offer free or low-cost ASL classes or Deaf mentor or coach services, where you can have a qualified Deaf adult come to your house for language services and guidance on deaf-specific parenting issues. Like deaf schools, service agencies can have other classes and services you'll want to use: Deaf camps, family events, educational advocacy, and legal help, and so on—look 'em up!

At your local university, community college, or adult-ed center: College programs are almost the only place to get systematic high-level ASL education, so if you're a real nerd, or if you want to level up quickly, they're the way to go. ASL interpreter or Deaf studies programs can be a great option, giving you the structure and support you need to pick up a new language. Plus, watching teenagers trying to rizz each other during class breaks is *hilarious*.

Personally, I need to flunk a few tests before I start taking my studies seriously, so ASL 1–4 at Berkeley City College was just the ticket. And I was lucky: BCC has a world-class ASL program, and I muddled my way through some excellent courses along with my wife. It wasn't always fun to leave school at 9:00 p.m. after working a full day, but a few semesters of pain were worth it in the long run.

College courses will naturally be more time intensive than other options, and the costs can vary. Community colleges are typically very affordable, but for our family, babysitting turned out to be the biggest financial challenge. Early intervention services can sometimes pay for tuition or childcare costs—see my chapter in EI later in the book.

And be careful—while these can be some of the best classes you can find, it's not always the case. Check with your local Deaf community if you can. As always, beware of programs with hearing teachers; Deaf teachers who use the language for themselves and "live the life" are the ones to get, if possible.

Inside the Internet: There has been a boom in online ASL teaching, and there are some very skilled instructors who will teach over Zoom. This is a huge advantage if you're caring for children or live far from other resources. One-on-one or group instruction from experienced Deaf teachers can be very affordable and a great education, but beware: there are a wide variety of hearing scammers and incompetents out there willing to take your money, or just your clicks, shoveling a lot of garbage and calling it "ASL." Some of these jokers have thousands of followers and put up a very slick front or associate with well-known online academies. Please be cautious before turning to hearing influencers or online teachers for your ASL, and if possible, cross-check or get references from other Deaf folks to make sure you're getting the real deal. And be aware that not every Deaf teacher or class will be a good fit for you, either! Shop around until you find someone you like working with.

But as I said, there are also plenty of websites, books, and video series that have good starter ASL for you and your kid, so you don't need to wait for classes to start learning and sharing with your baby. Check out suggestions at willfertman.com.

If *I'm* Not Going to Be Instantly Fluent in ASL, How Is My *Kid* Going to Learn It?

It takes a village, lots of YouTube, some Deaf role models, and a bunch of voices-off playdates to raise a deaf child. Again, current research indicates that hearing parents can learn alongside their babies at a pretty easy pace and support typical language development for their child.

But babies learn language everywhere they find it. While learning sign yourself is essential to this process, you're going to want to find additional ASL-fluent language models. Language models can be anyone—babysitters, playmates, teachers, mentors, family friends, and so on. Whoever and however you can expose your kid to fluent ASL, it's important to do it.

It's said that kids can pick up a language with a minimum of ten hours weekly of exposure, but more is always better, especially if this is your child's primary source of language. Daily interaction with fluent adults and kids is ideal. Having ASL-based childcare really helps: that can be an infant day program, a Deaf babysitter or nanny, or even a childcare swap with a Deaf parent. Check with Early Intervention, your local deaf school and deaf services agency, and check for Deaf childcare or Deaf community resources on social media, too. The *Schools, Preschools, Daycares, and Sitters* has more on this.

However, you might not find yourself in an ideal situation. Because deafness is fairly rare ("low incidence"), if you live in a rural area with a small Deaf population, or even just a state with shitty Early Intervention, you may have few choices. In these cases, you may be traveling far to find the Deaf events and going online to get that community exposure. That doesn't mean you shouldn't still learn ASL and expose your child as much as you can, but it does mean that there's a lot more homework, networking, and creative solutions you will need to explore. Fortunately, many more resources are now available online than even a few years ago.

Some families end up relocating to be close to services, particularly good deaf schools, but that's not always doable. If you're considering a move, please be careful: local school district regulations vary widely, so there's no guarantee that even if you move to the same town or city as a good deaf program, your child will be eligible for it under their rules. You'll want to do a lot of research to make sure you know the process involved—talk to parents and administrators at your target program / school, and at the local school district you're thinking of moving to before making the leap.

What Are Deaf Mentors or Deaf Coaches?

One great way to get ASL support for you and your child is a Deaf mentor or Deaf coach. There are mentor programs all over the country run by different entities—the SKI-HI Institute began the Deaf mentor training in the 1970s and has started programs in over twenty states, but there are independent local programs, too, run by schools, deaf services agencies, or early intervention. These programs pair new parents with trained Deaf adults who can answer questions and support parents and kids in their sign language learning. They are enormously valuable, and if you have one in your community, please take advantage of it.

Deaf adults are an amazing resource—they were deaf kids, after all, so they have insight for parents that goes way beyond teaching ASL. They know the ins and outs of deaf childhood, what's up in the local Deaf community, fun accessible events or organizations, and other hot tips. But a huge benefit from a mentor program isn't the explicit learning. Just knowing a Deaf adult can help soothe a lot of fears about what's in store for your kid. I remember bursting into tears the first time I met our family's Deaf mentor. Having this kind, smart, funny woman cooing over my baby boy was an overwhelming relief. I was so worried for my child's future, but here was a wonderful person who was like my child, the kind of person he could one day be. Parents need role models, too.

Will My Kid Become a Doctor?

Yes. This is my personal guarantee. Positions are also available for racecar driver, airplane mechanic, momfluencer, cartoonist, ballet dancer, lobster fisherman, lawyer, actor/model/whatever, research scientist, rap artist, carpenter, and e-sports streaming tycoon.

What Should I Do Next?

If you've got a deaf baby or toddler on your hands and you need a plan, here you go.

If you're still waiting for the doctors to get their shit together and give you a diagnosis:

In the United States, an official diagnosis of "hearing loss" can take a long time. You might get called back for multiple hearing tests of different sorts, possibly MRI or CAT scans as well. This can take months, but it's important to persevere and insist on getting it on paper as soon as possible. This is especially critical if you feel that your doctor or insurance agency is being slow or not responsive—some professionals don't take early childhood deafness as seriously as they should.

You may need a medical diagnosis to be eligible for free services like speech-language therapy, Deaf mentors, day programs, and so on via Early Intervention or Special Education services. Starting as soon as possible is key—without EI, you've got to find and pay for services on your own, and you'll be locked out of many opportunities. See the chapter *Audiograms and the "Hearing Loss" Diagnosis* for information on getting around this roadblock.

However, you don't need to wait for the doctors to catch up in order to start building your child's language skills and connecting with a supportive community. Go online and start ASL classes somewhere. If it turns out your baby isn't deaf, you still get to be the cool parents who can talk to their kid underwater. Also, get in touch with your local deaf school and deaf services agency—sometimes they're quite short-staffed, so you may need to be persistent. They have the most experience with the local scene and may have advice, educational programs, and recommendations for professionals who are hip to deaf children, which can also speed up the diagnostic phase. If there are local Deaf family events or playgroups, you may be able to attend or have other opportunities to connect with Deaf adults and the parents of deaf children.

If your kid has been identified as deaf and is under age three, but you're not enrolled in early intervention yet:

Besides ASL classes and finding your local Deaf community, you need to get in touch with your state's EI program and get enrolled. If your child was identified in the newborn screening at the hospital, or at an audiologist after that, EI should have already contacted you, but sometimes things don't happen the way they should. Early Intervention qualifies you for a lot of free educational and supportive services, and it's essential to help set up your kid's future education through the IFSP and IEP processes. In the United States, you can just Google your state's name plus "early intervention" to get a phone number or online form to register for EI on your own; this is known as *self-referral*.

If your kid is over the age of three but has just got identified as deaf:

You should start an IEP process. Contact your local school district's special education department to set it up, and don't take "no" or "504" for an answer. See if you can get a Deaf educational advocate from your local deaf services agency or another organization to help with this.

If you're already enrolled in early intervention or special education and already learning ASL:

Relax. Please. It was nerve-wracking for us to have a deaf baby, but you're going to be ok. Looking back, I wish I could have taken some more time to just play with Oscar and his brother and appreciate my family.

There will be a lot of discussions regarding hearing technology coming up, but those you'll mostly handle in the audiologist's or doctor's offices. In the meantime, keep learning ASL and find a Deaf mentor or Deaf community group you can participate in. Sign with your baby, learn some nursery rhymes and baby books, and please, enjoy your time.

The next thing is to start preparing for your Individual Family Service Plan (IFSP) or Individualized Education Program (IEP). This is the master record of everything that's going on with your kid, and the key document that lays out all the therapy and accommodations the state is going to supply. Check out the later chapter during your 3:00 a.m. feeding; I guarantee it's riveting.

Anything Else?

My website, willfertman.com, has resources for learning ASL, finding Deaf-savvy professional mentors, helpful community organizations, book recommendations, sources for cute baby clothes, and other stuff. The whole rest of the book is the nitty-gritty.

Go get some sleep.

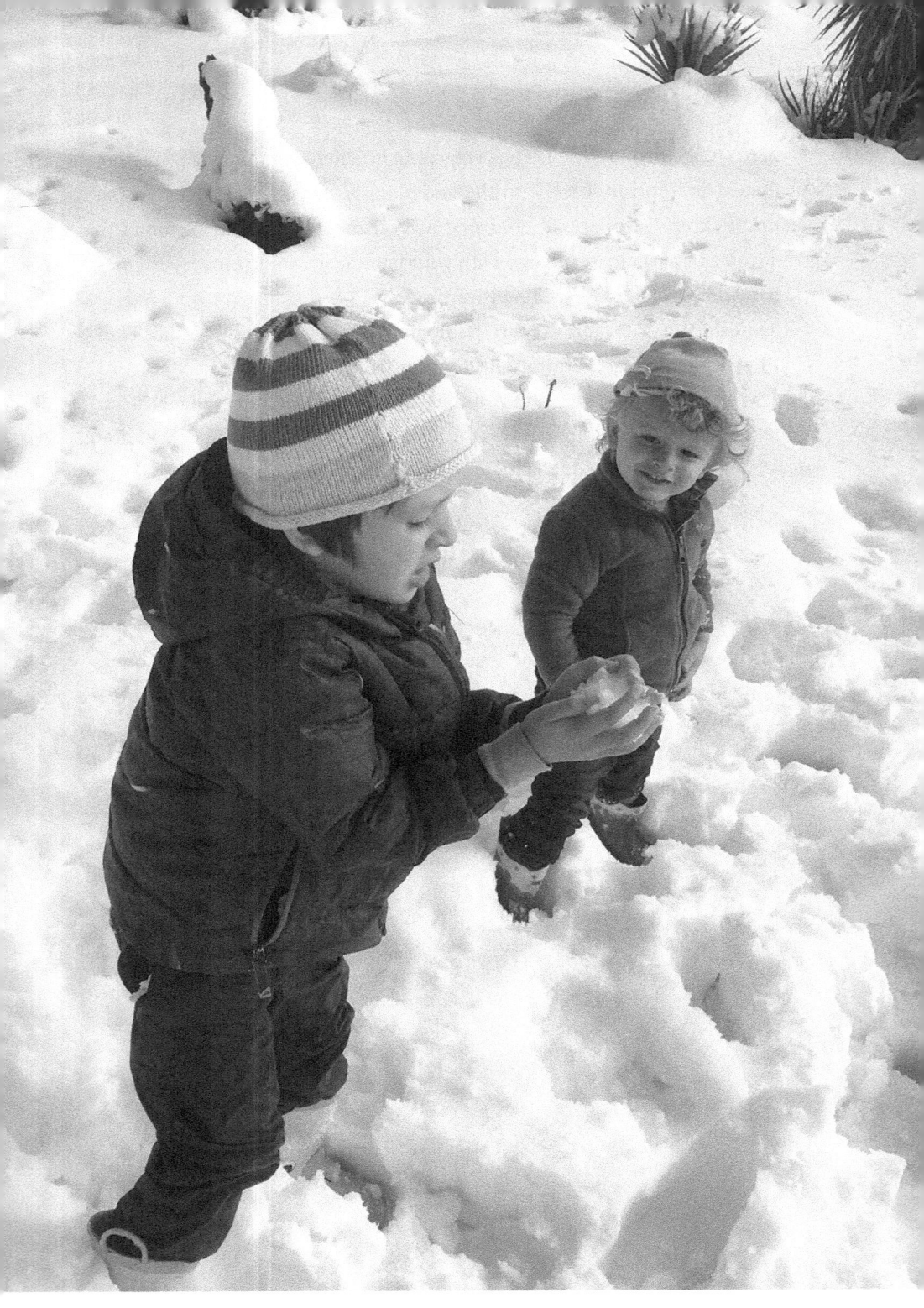

Will Fertman, 2025

2

Day to Day with Your Deaf Baby

Having a baby is a lot. For a hearing parent, having a deaf baby is a lot more—more appointments, more medical procedures, more classes, more weird social pressure, more sleepless nights. The first year of Oscar's life was especially stressful, as we fretted, studied, and slowly changed gears to become a bilingual family.

But now that he's past kindergarten and doing great, do I cherish all the late nights sweating over his IFSP, agonizing whether to get him CIs, or staring into the Internet abyss, sick with worry? I do not. I *do* remember the time I took Oscar and his brother down to the pier for dinner. Leo hid in the basket under the stroller. I put the food on top of Oscar, and Leo grabbed sushi off his belly as we walked. People stared, but we had a blast.

It's easy to lose sight of the fact that our children are not problems to be solved; they're little people to be played with, cared for, and adored. Unless your child has very serious medical needs, most of your time is going to be spent outside of doctors' offices and therapy sessions, feeding them, playing with them, changing their diapers, taking them on walks, and so on.[1] Long, slow days, where your child is nobody's responsibility but your own.

---

[1] And if your child *does* need a high level of medical care, the times when you can play, cuddle, and connect outside of a medical context are even *more* precious.

This section is devoted to the things you can do on your own to support your kid and their siblings, have a good time with them and the rest of your family, while making sure they get the language exposure and full inclusion they deserve.

How to Sign with a Baby

Babies, hearing or deaf, *love* sign language. There's nothing more gratifying than the way their little eyes light up when they recognize you're communicating with them. *And babies do not care how good or fluent you are,* so they will be your best practice partners. Any time you and your child are together, put your hands up and get to it!

There's no wrong way to do it, and no special moment to begin; start signing whatever you can as soon as you can. Use whatever ASL words, sentences, or rhymes you've already learned—and fill in the rest with gestures and mimes. Point out objects and name them. Ask if they want milk. Tell them it's time to change their diaper. It's helpful to learn some baby-oriented vocabulary first—you'll have a lot more opportunities to chat if you know the signs for BATH and BOTTLE, but if you happen to know the sign for PSYCHOTHERAPIST, and a psychotherapist walks by, throw it in. Children learn all kinds of language all the time and will be watching you for clues on how to communicate.

While the following are tips on how to use sign with your child, I just want to repeat that to actually learn *ASL, you'll want to find a Deaf teacher of some kind.*

Get Low and Close

The first time I saw a fluent signer—a child of Deaf adults (CODA)—interact with my kid, she dropped straight to the rug and got up in his face. He loved it.

Typical infants are nearsighted; get close and you'll notice their attention zap straight to you. In the stroller, during tummy time, when they're in a sling or backpack, or a high chair, you've got a captive audience. Scootch up and get your hands in there.

Go Big

Just like you'd exaggerate baby talk, you can slow down your signs slightly and make them nice and big for an infant. Don't go overboard—as a beginner you're already signing very slowly, but be deliberate give it some rhythm if you can. Watching native ASL nursery rhymes from skilled signers (like in the Hands Land television show) can be very helpful to get a sense of what "Mommy-style" signing looks like.

Ham It Up

ASL relies on *big* facial expressions to get your point across, and babies are drawn to that. All the emotional inflection you would put into your speaking voice, you've got to put onto your face and body. When you sign MILK, show how delicious the milk is. When you sign TIGER, be fierce, like a tiger. Sign HAPPY and give your biggest smile, and SAD with your saddest frown.

Sign on Their Body

This is a fun method of playing with language that doesn't really have an equivalent in English. It can be done in two ways. If your baby is in your lap or otherwise facing away from you, sign as if your hands were theirs. Hold your five-hand to their forehead to sign DAD, or touch your two-hand next to their eye while signing LOOK, and so on. Not only is this fun, it's super useful with visual kids, who sometimes prefer to be facing out toward the world. Signing on their bodies in this way allows you to keep talking to them even while they're looking away from you.

On the other hand, if your baby is facing you, you can "travel" a sign, so DAD might start on your forehead and zip over to touch theirs in the same spot. Or a sign like MOUSE (an index finger twitching your nose) might start on your nose and scurry down your chest and up their body to their nose, like a real mouse. Both techniques help develop your baby's sense of how the language "occurs" on their body, part of a process of language learning called *phonological awareness*.

Sign Your ABCs and 123s

The manual alphabet is probably the first ASL "song" you're going to learn by heart. Not only is this just a quality nursery rhyme, the letters of the ASL alphabet, along with the signs for numbers, are used as handshapes in many other words—the F handshape is used to sign IMPORTANT, the 5 handshape is used to sign GRANDMA, and so on. Distinguishing handshapes is another aspect of phonological awareness, which will build your baby's overall language skills. There are at least fifty handshapes in ASL, and the alphabet and basic numbers cover more than half. So whenever there's a spare moment, count what you see and bust out your ABCs.

Fingerspell

While we're on the topic of letters, you should know that ASL sometimes depicts words by spelling them out letter by letter. Fingerspelling is an integral part of ASL, and you should use it whenever it's appropriate—people's names, businesses, or other proper nouns, and ASL words that are typically fingerspelled like BANK.

Don't worry if your child is too young to read. Even if they don't know their alphabet yet, they're learning to see the whole movement of your hand as a single word, and kids will very quickly learn the fingerspelled words for the things they like. Before my son turned two, he recognized fingerspelled vocabulary like BUS, PARK, and PICKLE, and knew the fingerspelled names of all his favorite people: Leo, Carrie, Caitlin, Emily, Barrett, Sarah . . .

Studies have shown that fingerspelling is a key bridge to literacy for deaf kids; at first, they only see the *movement envelope*, but slowly they discover the letters embedded inside. That becomes a clue to help them recognize those letters on paper.

Use a Lot of Classifiers

In ASL, *classifiers* are like little puppets you make with your hands to describe the physical world. A downward two-handshape is a person that can walk, jump, or do a little dance. A three-handshape on its side is a car that you can zoom around, park, or crash, and a five-handshape can be an ocean wave, a fire, or a splat of ketchup on your face!

Classifiers are an essential part of the language and incredibly practical; they let you pack in so much information that ASL descriptions of events or objects are often more thorough and precise than English equivalents. But they're *very* different from English, so you'll want to remind yourself to use classifiers when you're telling stories, giving instructions, or describing events to your child. It takes practice.

Kids "get" classifiers and will eventually start playing with them and telling their own stories with their hands. It's adorable.

Be Playful

Generally, just play with your hands, be expressive, and don't be shy. If you're stuck for a word or want to get goofy, throw in some gestures or mimes, too. While gestures aren't language, they are a part of ASL storytelling, and research shows that gesture helps deaf kids connect concepts and help bridge gaps when parents don't know specific words. Sign language has a lot of opportunities to put on a show, and kids learn best when they're playing, so the more fun and exuberant you can be with it, the better.

Those are all the do's. There's one big don't, though:

Don't Sign and Talk at the Same Time

ASL sentences can have a different structure than English. Deaf artist Christine Sun Kim compares English to playing a melody on a piano with just one hand, while ASL is like playing two-handed chords. English sentences are linear, one word following another, while ASL sentences give a lot of information simultaneously. Because of this, signing and talking at the same time—officially called *SimCom*—is going to trip you up. Just imagine trying to speak English and write Russian all at once.

Studies have shown that when SimCom'ing, English will tend to dominate your conversation, while your ASL will start to fall apart, becoming slow and incoherent. This is true even for skillful signers, but for a beginner, it will be a big roadblock not just for clear communication with your baby, but also for you learning correct ASL. There are plenty of teachers out there who were taught to SimCom and will try to teach you the same way, but it's an outmoded method that's been shown to do more harm than good.

This doesn't mean that you won't ever see SimCom "in the wild," or do it occasionally yourself, but it's done as a fudge, often for brief statements or announcements. If you've got a hearing/Deaf household like ours, there are just some moments when you've got to make sure everyone's on the same page. SimComming STOP is pretty common, followed by GET OFF THE ROOF. But beyond emergencies, if you've got something to say in both ASL and English, separate the languages. First sign it, then say it (or vice versa).

This separation also applies if you need to explain or define a word that your kid knows in one language but not the other. It's called the sandwich technique: first use the familiar word or sign, then the new one, then the familiar one again: APPLE / "apple" / APPLE.

Also note that it's common to quietly speak or *mouth* single English words while you're signing ASL. Sometimes this is used to add emphasis or clarify a sign with multiple meanings, or it's just because you're a native English speaker and your brain comes up with the spoken word first. **Mouthing is totally fine, and it is not SimCom**; when you mouth, you're not trying to marry two different sentence structures together, just match a word or two here and there, and it's generally not an impediment to expressing or learning clear ASL.

Baby Signs Back

Because they learn to control their hands before they can control their lips, tongue, and voicebox, babies with typical motor development—deaf or not—are able to sign long before they can speak. I've seen incredibly tiny infants signing MILK and MOM. Our deaf son's first word came around five months old; he was lying back in his stroller, looking up into the leaves, holding his arm straight up and waving an open hand in the air, the sign for TREE. So, if your kid was identified as deaf early, and you were able to start sign with them, you will have major bragging rights on the playground.

But don't sweat it if your child isn't signing when they're still in the womb. Although keeping an eye on language development is absolutely essential if you're the hearing parent of a deaf kid, remember that signing is just like talking, walking, or potty training; there's a developmental spectrum for it, and some kids may arrive earlier or later. As long as your child has access to language and fluent language models, you're on the right path.

California's LEAD-K milestones state that a deaf child should have one to three expressive signs before one year old, but there are many other developmental markers to look out for. The milestones are a solid guide to deaf baby language development, even if you don't live in Cali, and I've included a link to them at willfertman.com, but discuss your kid's progress with your child's SLP and ToD as well.

Babblin' Fingles

Before your child starts signing, they will babble; this comes at around four to six months, and it's a key developmental step all children use to build their basic language skills. Deaf babies will start by babbling with their mouths, just like hearing babies, but that may taper off if they don't have the residual hearing to get feedback from their own voices. However, babies who are surrounded by sign language will also start to babble with their hands and make little flicks and gestures that don't mean anything on their own, but which are deadly cute and which are building up to making full signs. Keep an eye out for them. Words are soon to follow.

Baby Talk, ASL Style

Babies sign the way babies speak—not always clearly, and not always consistently. Most kids can't pull off complex handshapes or nail a sign's proper positioning, and they will not perform on command. The sign for MOM is supposed to land on the chin, but if it hits their cheek, that's just extra sweet. Don't feel bad if you have trouble spotting your kid's first attempts—if you're a beginner, it's tough to notice the difference between random flailing, purposeful babbling, and a word. This is an area where it helps to have a Deaf person involved, as a native signer will have an easier time recognizing and decoding cute 'n clumsy signs.

Once you do spot a word, make sure you respond! Copy it, bring them the thing they signed, let them know they did a good job, just be enthusiastic and communicative. Positive feedback is what your child needs to start learning language.

Talky Talk, Bilingual Style

Babies who have access to spoken language through residual hearing or devices will start picking up English, too, and those CA LEAD-K / SB 210 milestones work equally well for sign and spoken language. Your kid's speech will probably lag sign by a certain amount just because of motor development and the relative access to sound that your kid may have. Also, keep in mind that bilingual babies tend to start a little more slowly in each language. That's ok—*collectively* they should be keeping pace.

The trick is distinguishing between global and individual language development. Global development is really looking at the underlying brain development—not just their ability to use one language, but their ability to use languages as a whole. For bilingual kids, this means that you're taking all their abilities in all their languages into account when you're measuring their developmental progress. For instance, when you're tracking a bilingual child's vocabulary for this purpose, you would count all the words they recognize or express in ASL and in English, and add them together to get a total count.

This is different from measuring their individual language development. As you'll read in the chapter on IFSP and IEPs, goals and services for English, ASL, and other languages should be listed separately and never combined. As kids get older, if they're getting fluent exposure to both languages, their individual abilities in different languages should progress, but it won't happen at the same speed, and they will need different levels of support, so you'll have to track them individually.

In fact, it's common for bilingual kids to pick a favorite expressive language and stick to that one under most circumstances. My son is a big talker, and if he's with us, he'll speak English, regardless of whether we're signing with him or not. It's pretty common for deaf kids in hearing families to do this, so don't get frustrated if your child decides they only want to talk or if they only want to sign. Keep exposing them to both languages and keep learning ASL yourself. Kids' needs will change over time, so even if you have a very English-y two-year-old today, you may find yourself with a very ASL-y six-year-old. In Oscar's case, while he's very talky at home, he's also perfectly happy to sign his way through his deaf school and will shush me if I accidentally say something to him on campus. "Dad—this place is signing only!"

Dividing the Day's Language

Remember that kids need at least ten hours weekly of exposure to have a shot at acquiring a given language, and if English is *your* first language, you'll tend to use it more, unless you've got a system in place. A useful technique is finding those times of day when you always use sign versus when you always use spoken language. And since children are creatures of habit, it helps *them* figure out when to switch languages if there are concrete rules for when and where you use one language over another.

For our family, it worked best for us to have signed meal times when we would play games and chat in ASL with Oscar and his brother. Added to this were the many situations like bath times or naps when my kid's CIs would come off, plus any time we were spending around other Deaf adults. But the particular mix changed many times over the course of his childhood as schedules shifted, and his access to signing role models changed. Having a system helps, but don't be afraid to redo the rules.

Getting Attention

One of the big challenges in having a deaf child is getting their attention when they're focused on something else. Kids are often (and rightly) lost in their own world; they're learning machines, and there's an infinite amount to learn, so it can be hard to pull them away from whatever experiment they're doing. Studies show that deaf children take in more information from their peripheral vision than hearing kids do and process visual data faster. But that might not be obvious when you're frantically windmilling your arms, trying to stop them from dropping your wallet into the toilet.

Deaf culture has a standard set of tactics for getting attention that are (sometimes) effective with young children. It's good to practice them anyway, as you'll want to use them with the Deaf adults you meet.

The wave: The obvious choice for children and Deaf adults. Make an expectant face and do a little wave. It's always worth a try, although it's generally the least successful tactic with my kid. Sometimes, if you're in a sunny environment, you can get your shadow to fall in their field of view, too, so that helps. A homestyle variation on this is **the fan:** if my guy is close but out of reach, I've found it effective to grab a book or another flat object and actually move some air. It works for us, but it has no currency in Deaf culture.

The shoulder tap: When your child has their back to you, but you're close, you can try firmly tapping their shoulder or upper arm to get their attention. The official "Deaf tap" is once or twice on the shoulder with the tips of a flat, bent hand, woodpecker style. With your kid, you'll be tempted to tap whatever body part is within reach, but for Deaf adults, the rules of contact are strict: no touching anything but the shoulder, no grabbing or directing the person, and no Cheeto dust on the fingers.

The floor stomp: If you're not standing on concrete or wearing stilettos, stomping on the floor can be a good way to remotely signal your kid. Some gentle table-pounding can have the same effect if you're sitting down. It can feel awkward—shaking the room is a social taboo in the hearing world—but it works and is perfectly polite in Deaf company.

The light switch flick: The preferred tactic in our house. Turning the lights off and on can be effective at getting a visual baby's attention and is useful when they're across the room, or if you don't want to annoy the downstairs neighbors with a stomp. This is a standard approach in Deaf culture; Deaf households frequently use flashing overhead lights for doorbells, phone calls, and other alerts. Viva Thomas Edison!

Not recommended:

Yelling: Just no. I mean, you're a parent. Sooner or later, you *will* yell, but don't get into the habit of yelling for kids' attention: remember that louder doesn't always mean clearer for a deaf child. And don't yell at Deaf adults. At all.

Throwing stuff (soft or otherwise): Everyone eventually uses this at one point, too, but it's not a great habit to get into. Deaf adults sometimes chuck balls of paper or other innocuous weapons to get each other's attention, but you've got to know somebody pretty well to pelt them with a stuffie.

Danger Alert! AKA, Sign Names

Do not give your baby an ASL sign name.

Now that you've been warned, you will want to get your baby a sign name;[2] let's face it, fingerspelling "Augustine Xavier Gabriel the 3rd" is going to get tedious. But sign names are a place where you'll run headfirst into sacred Deaf cultural traditions, so you need to be prepared.

Here's the deal: your name in ASL is just your name, fingerspelled. Mine is W-I-L-L-I-A-M. Even if you've given your kid a hippie name like Star, it's still just S-T-A-R, spelled out letter by letter. You should use this name for your child when first introducing them to a new person, and you should teach it to your kid so they recognize and answer to it.

Sign names are different: they're a unique shorthand in ASL that you can use for someone you know or someone famous instead of fingerspelling. They are more like, *but not the same as*, nicknames in English and are a unique feature of Deaf culture. There are a lot of rules as to what makes a good sign name and how they are given and used, but the most important rule of all is this:

Sign Names Can Only Be Given by Members of the Deaf Community

Whether that's family, friends, teachers, or other folks, a sign name has got to come from a Deaf person. This might seem unfair to us hearing parents; we get to name our own kids, right? But giving sign names is a deeply held cultural

---

[2] Also, "name signs"—either one works.

value in the Deaf community, rooted in the ways children were brought together by residential schools or were raised in generational Deaf families. It's one of the great Deaf traditions and you've got to respect it.

Keep in mind that you've already named your baby in ASL—that's their fingerspelled name, and that's the one that most people, Deaf and hearing, will know them by for the rest of their lives. The sign name isn't that name, it's something different that grows out of their relationship with their peers and community. Making an end run around this tradition signals that you don't value Deaf culture, and by extension, the people included in that culture—like your own child.

But besides showing respect, the "Deaf only" rule protects you in a very practical way: **having fluent signers give a sign name eliminates the possibility of accidentally naming your kid TOILET and subsequently getting the sign for TOILET tattooed on your body.** Hang around parents' forums long enough and you'll find some truly unfortunate stories. Save yourself a lot of heartache and Deaf-Internet infamy and leave sign names to the pros.

Hilariously, there's no *lower* age limit for Deaf people to give sign names, so be prepared for your kid to eventually start handing them out to others, like uncle GROUCHY BEARD, for instance.

Not Everyone Gets a Sign Name

Sign names aren't initiation ceremonies. Although they are one connection your child (or you) might have to the Deaf community, having one doesn't mean you're in or out of the club. Especially if they have a short or easy-to-fingerspell name, your child may just never end up with a sign name, and that's fine.

Sign Names Don't Necessarily Contain Awesome Secret Meanings

You might want to have some beautiful, aspirational meaning behind your child's sign name, but that's not how they work. Sign names are drawn from a lot of sources; they might have an insight into your child's personality, or be related to a physical feature or a habit they have, or a piece of clothing they often wear, or be based on their name or initials, or they might be entirely arbitrary. My younger son's sign name comes from the word SKEPTICAL. One of his friend's sign names is based on the *last* two letters of his name. Another friend has a sign name that's just a gesture she'd make as a baby, and has no meaning in ASL at all. When they do have a meaning, sign names aren't always flattering. Politicians in particular are often subject to very insulting ones, incorporating words like LIAR or classifiers for TOUPEE.

Sign Names Change

Sign names can change over time or in a new social environment. Your kid may end up with a name at school or among their friends that's different from the one you use at home. My son's sign name has begun to mutate as his friends and teachers use it, moving away from the one he was originally given. As he grows, he might get a completely different one for any number of reasons. It's all good.

Getting Started With a Sign Name

If you want to have some say in your child's sign name, let the Deaf adults in their life know. If your child has a Deaf family member, mentor, or teacher, they can consult with you to come up with something good. *Remember that there are more rules about sign names than the ones I've just listed*: please follow their lead.[3]

Also be aware that while some Deaf folks are very serious about giving sign names, others might not care much or feel comfortable doing it, especially if they don't know your kid well. Just be cool; it's not a secret handshake, and nobody's obligated to give, or have, a sign name.

If you're new to all this and don't have Deaf adults to help you out yet, you can still use something safe and temporary as a placeholder. Fingerspelling is always correct, so if you named your kid Ed or Liz, you're all set. If your child's

---

[3] If you're really curious, Deaf YouTuber Rogan Shannon has a video about sign names from an insider's POV.

name is something longer and you want to keep things simple, the first letter of your kid's name tapped on your heart usually works. Let people know that this is just what you're doing for now and be ready to let it go if or when a proper sign name appears.

Baby Care Basics

Caring for a deaf baby is 95 percent identical to caring for a hearing child. Here's how to tackle the rest.

Bedtime, Sleep, and Associated Misery

This is a good news/bad news situation. The good news is that being deaf doesn't really affect your baby's ability to sleep per se. Some deaf-linked syndromes like CHARGE can have impacts on sleep, but simply not being able to hear isn't the problem. Having a deaf kid can even spoil you; you'll get very cavalier about loud conversations, music, and vacuuming during naptime. The bad news is, they're still a baby, so no matter what, sleep ain't guaranteed.

If you've already gone through sleep training with a hearing child, my advice will be very familiar, and I would recommend starting with whatever approach you liked and that worked before. Every baby is individual, so you'll need to experiment anyway. Some kids are the kings of naps, others are colicky nightmares. And just like hearing children, deaf children's needs will change: a good sleeper at six months might have awful sleep regression at eight months, and then be a champion again until they're three, then fall off the wagon, and so on.

So there isn't a magic bullet for getting a deaf infant to sleep, but being aware of what your baby's senses are like and what they're paying attention to is going to help you troubleshoot when you're trying to squeeze a couple more minutes out of the night.

Setting Up the Nursery

> We spent a lot of time stumbling in the dark. If I could do it again, I'd get night vision goggles.
>
> my wife

Deaf children are visual. Thinking about their bedrooms means thinking about light, lines of sight, and other visual factors. When you're putting a baby down, look at the room from their perspective—is something blocking their view of you? Are there beams of light coming through from outside, or another room? Does your kid see your shadow when you move past the crib? Is there a blinking smoke detector or bright digital clock in their field of view? These things might be distracting or stimulating when your child is trying to settle down.

Touch, temperature, and vibration are other sensations to consider: do your footsteps shake the crib when you walk by? Does opening the door change the air pressure in the room? Do you have a dishwasher, toilet, or clothes dryer whose vibrations can be felt in the nursery?

This does more than create the right environment for sleeping. Since your kid will be looking and feeling for information, you can use those visual and tactile cues to help communicate with them. So if the lights are off, you might stomp a little on the floor to signal that you're still nearby. Or you might always close the blinds at naptime so your baby can see a stripy shadow on the wall and know it's time to settle down. Babies thrive on routine, so the more signals you can send to them about what they should be doing, the easier it will be to get them into a groove.

As a newborn, Oscar was up every two to three hours—no surprises there. But between six and twelve months, he was a reasonable sleeper. He needed a very dark room: blackout curtains helped, and with that darkness, he could get through some long stretches overnight. But then something changed, and suddenly he would be up and crying constantly. Slowly it dawned on us that our visual baby was not comforted by the dark anymore. If he woke in total darkness, he was starting to panic. So we began to keep the curtains open to let some light in from the street, and if he briefly came awake, he could often get himself back down.

Now that he's five, it's different again. He's mobile and wants to be with us all the time. If he wakes in the night and gets a clue that we're awake too, he'll run straight to our bed. This means that we've got to be careful about light—the bathroom is next to his room, so if you want to keep him in bed, you've got to close the door before turning on the light. Otherwise, he'll see the glow in his bedroom and sneak out to party with us.

Soothing

Soothing a deaf baby is a little different. A late-night wakeup means working in the dark, and holding the kid in your arms means not always having hands available to sign. Depending on your child's residual hearing, that may not matter—you're right up close, in a quiet environment, and can sing or speak very near your baby's ears. And maybe your child just likes holding and rocking, and feeling the vibrations of your body while you sing or talk. On the other hand, this may be the job for a small nightlight or closet/hallway light that can make you visible without bombarding your kid with sleep-obliterating illumination.

One thing that's worked well for us is touch. When our profoundly deaf guy was an infant in a co-sleeper next to the bed, I would often reach over and just lay my hand on his chest to help calm him. Having that touch frequently helped him get back down at night. We also sometimes used tactile signing. Hold your baby in a position that's comfortable and use one or both hands to give them a little song by touch. For lack of anything better, I signed the ABCs on his back a lot, but you can fingerspell their names, or sign MOMMY ILY gently on their chin and chest—whatever works and helps them get into a groove. And don't forget that they can still feel your voice through your body, so while the sound of your singing might not reach them, if you hold them close, the vibrations of your voice and rocking of your body will.

Hearing Devices in the Crib

If your baby wears hearing aids, BAHAs, or cochlear implants, you can try taking them off before putting them down for bed and integrating that into the sleep routine. Lowering the overall stimulation can be an advantage when you're trying to get them to settle. This may or may not work; ultimately, you will need to follow your child's lead. My son liked falling asleep with his CIs on—and with music playing!—for a long time, although I always took them off once he was down.

Please don't leave your child's hearing devices on all night. I've heard of some audiologists recommending it in case of a late-night wakeup, but CIs and HAs aren't actually meant to be worn 24/7. They can irritate ears or the scalp, and leaving them in the crib unattended is a choking hazard if your kid gets them into their mouth, let alone the issue of loose batteries to swallow. Yikes.

This is not only a safety issue. Giving your child some "deaf time" is key to helping them understand and be comfortable in their own bodies and with their own experiences. These days, my son actually takes his CIs off as a signal that he's ready for bed. The quiet helps him relax, and we can sign together when he needs to communicate at night.

> Requiring children to sleep with their implants or hearing aids gives them the message that they cannot be Deaf, and increases the likelihood of panic when their tech fails. It's social conditioning that they are not enough, which becomes hard to break as adults, because they will believe that it is not "safe" to be Deaf. Nothing can be further from the truth.
>
> This is not an anti-tech statement, but rather an encouragement to set healthy boundaries, and to foster confidence in our children that they are enough.
>
> Professor Bee Vicars, Deaf ASL educator

Feeding

You'll be doing a lot of this, and mealtime is one of the prime moments for sharing language. Whether you're nursing, feeding them from a bottle, or on to solids, always ask your kid those rhetorical mom questions, which are an important part of language development: "Are you hungry? Do you want more? Does that taste good?" This is also a likely place for your child's first signs to appear—food is the ultimate motivator.

As your child starts eating in a high chair or booster seat, you'll find it's a great format for ASL. Your baby is seated upright at eye level—a captive audience! All those "Here comes the airplane!" things are perfect to sign and gives you a chance to work on your classifiers, your colors, food names, emotions, and more. Mealtime is also a great time to share books or play language games for the same reason. Check out *Reading to Your Child* and *Kitchen Table ASL Games* for more.

Bathtime

Bath time is another good no-technology moment. It's a chance for your kid to "power down," enjoy their sensory world, and build their comfort with their own deaf bodies. Bath time is a major moment for language sharing, too: naming their different body parts in ASL, playing with bath toys, and talking about sensations like HOT, COLD, SLIPPERY, and so on.

One word of warning: hard surfaces in the tub + the usual "don't wash my hair" screaming x child with no volume control = *loud* bathtimes. Even if they're not upset, the sound-amplifying nature of bathrooms can encourage deaf kids to pump up the volume and experiment with their residual hearing. Earplugs (for you) aren't out of the question.

Diapers and Potties

Barring additional disabilities, deaf kids don't poop different, so diapering is the same as with a hearing child. You might want to hang a mirror near the changing table because visual infants can sometimes get worried if a parent ducks out of sight for a second to grab a wipe. It can also help your kid know what's happening by allowing them a view of themselves; blowout disposal and ASL are both two-handed activities.

Potty training deaf toddlers is a lot like sleep training—there's no magic method, but if you've done it with a hearing child, start with what worked and be ready to modify your tactics. Whether your kid uses ASL, spoken English, or both, training is not going to run smoothly without open channels of communication. You've got to keep encouraging them and have the language skills to explain what can be a dauntingly complex process to a young child. Parent-oriented ASL courses like ASL at Home can help with specific vocabulary and sentence structure.

Because *executive function*[4] is tied to language acquisition, language-deprived kids can struggle with potty training. If your child was late-identified

---

[4] The set of skills that helps children plan and carry out complicated tasks.

as deaf and is in the process of catching up, you might find that they need more time to get it. The kid is going to lead the way, but in general, it's language before toilet. Picture books are always a help, especially when they have concrete, step-by-step illustrations. Don't be afraid to bring your child into the bathroom with you, and potentially even give them an in-person demonstration. As parents of toddlers soon learn, whether your child is language deprived or not, the ability to shit in their presence can be a critical parenting skill.

Shopping

Shopping for cute stuff is half the fun of having a kid! Feel free to xerox this section and send it to all grandparents, aunties, and other well-wishers (and send them a link to willfertman.com, which has links to Deaf companies and designers for sourcing).

Toys

Like sleep and potty training, toys are going to be very individual. Baby Oscar had a passionate and complicated relationship with a plastic banana mobile hanging over his crib. Focusing on visual and tactile experiences is going to be helpful, though: night light projectors or light-up rattles, mirrors and optical toys, colorful objects and mobiles, fun-to-touch textures and vibrating doohickies are all great ways to engage their senses. Just be aware that wooden spoons and keyrings may be just as popular. Lay in a supply of baby board books, too, because it's never too early.

Some kids will appreciate sound-based toys that they can either feel the vibrations from or hear with their residual hearing. One of the best early toys for our son was a Bluetooth speaker in the shape of a Rubik's Cube that lit up when music was playing. He loved holding it, watching the lights flash, and feeling the rhythm of the music playing through it, especially with something bassy jiggling his innards. Noisemakers like drums and xylophones with a lot of reverb are great, too. Just keep in mind that YOU will also have to hear whatever noise they're making, and that their preference might be for skull-crackingly loud sounds, so choose carefully.

ASL Toys

There are a small number of ASL-oriented toys available; in particular, ASL alphabet blocks or tiles are a must-have. And while there are some quality products out there being made by companies and individuals, be careful. Hearing makers sometimes get the signs wrong for one reason or another, so whenever possible, buy from a Deaf shop.

You can also occasionally find teddy bears and dolls with glove-hands you can slip into so they can sign, as well as stuffed animals or dolls with hearing devices if your child wears one. You can also just DIY devices with a sharpie or a little bit of modeling clay. Spider-Man toys are popular too, because he's always making the I LOVE YOU / ILY sign with his hand.

ASL Baby Clothes and Nursery Decorations

There are a LOT of cute baby clothes out there with ASL graphics and Deaf-positive messages. I LOVE YOU / ILY shirts and onesies are practically mandatory, but there are more creative designs available to show your pride. We loved our OCTOPUS t-shirts from artist Jena Floyd, and Douglas Ridloff's "Deaf Vibe" shirts were the hottest thing last year.

Be warned that clothing with the ILY sign on it (or other "hearing loss isn't for wimps" stuff) is often produced by hearing companies with no connection to the Deaf community. Worse, hearing designers sometimes rip off the best stuff from Deaf designers, so check out the business profile before buying. Language Priority is a good Deaf-owned business to start with, but there are many others.

While you're shopping for clothes, you can find some ASL posters, calendars, or other decorations for the kid's room (or if you're at our house, the dining room). At a minimum, you gotta get an alphabet poster, but there are different designs out there showing animal signs, handshapes, and all sorts of different cute graphics. 58 Creativity is a good source for these.

Something that might be helpful for both you and your kid is labeling kits or flashcards that you can stick on different objects around the house to remind you of their ASL signs. As always, beware of hearing makers and stay away from "baby sign" products that might not be the real deal.

Your Accessible Home

As your child grows and starts getting mobile, there are a number of things you can do to make your apartment or house more deaf-friendly. While they're not absolutely necessary for an infant or toddler, making these changes alongside general childproofing work means that your kid can more naturally take part in family life, and you won't have to think about them later. When looking for specialty items like visual fire alarms, Diglo, the deaf hardware store, should be your first stop.

Visual doorbells: There are lots of models in lots of price ranges—some that have separate signal lights and chimes, and some that can be connected to existing lights to make them flash when the button is pushed. There are also *loud as hell* doorbells available for people with more residual hearing, but I don't recommend that solution in a mixed hearing/deaf household.

Visual smoke and carbon monoxide alarms: Alarms that have attached strobe lights for warnings along with the usual beeping can be a little expensive and fussy to install. The greater power demands of a strobe mean that they usually run on wall current rather than battery power and need to be put up by a professional. Because of this, the Red Cross, local fire departments, or deaf service agencies sometimes have programs to help out financially—check in your area. Otherwise, you'll need to buy the systems yourself and pay an electrician to wire it up. Because it's a critical safety tool, this is one area where you won't want to skimp.

Clearing sight lines: reducing visual clutter will help you and your child communicate, and it will help them see more of what's going on in your home. This is especially important at the kitchen table or any other place where the family meets for meals and discussion; get rid of centerpieces, vases, ketchup bottles, or other sight-blocking tchochkies. In family areas, see if you can keep the middle spaces open, so your kid can crawl or toddle around but not lose sight of you. Hanging a couple of mirrors can also help with visual contact and communication, or if you're really feeling your Norm Abram, you can knock out some walls to make that open plan kitchen/dining room you've always dreamed of.[5]

---

[5] Deaf architecture and design is a real field with fascinating insights into the ways Deaf folks live and communicate. You can find a lot of information about it online at organizations like World Deaf Architecture and Deaf Architecture Front.

Subtitles are go: Set all TVs and screens to closed captioning by default. Doesn't matter if your child is too young to read.

Lights: Make sure every room has good lighting—if it's dim, think about adding a second floor lamp or other indirect/shaded light to the room rather than just swapping out the overhead bulb for something brighter. It can help boost the overall light levels without blowing out your eyeballs. Also, think about adding light switches in areas near doorways for convenient flicking—the best way to get your kid's attention, IMO.

Going Out

Getting out of the house is hard when you've got a baby, but my God, a little sunlight and fresh air do wonders when you're chained to the cradle.

General Principles for Leaving the House

Plan for access and inclusion. Before you leave, give yourself a minute to think about how you're going to communicate with your child, how they're going to communicate with others, and what kind of access they'll need to participate in the event. Going to the park, just you and the babe? All you might need is a ball and applesauce. Going to a windy beach? Maybe leave the hearing aids safe at home and just sign. Family reunion? You may want an interpreter there so your kid can talk with his cousins, or an FM system or Bluetooth mic to zap conversations directly into his hearing devices. The answers will be different depending on your kid, their age, and where you're going. But a little forethought will go a long way.

Keep in mind that there are some outings that are impossible with hearing children but are awesome places to bring your deaf kids: Oscar loved the ultra-loud hip-hop exhibit at the Oakland Museum when he was eighteen months old and went back twice! ::*boom the bass*::

Strollers, Carriers, and Car Seats

When thinking about deaf infant transport, use the same concepts for baby movers that you use for cribs: think visually, and imagine how your kid is using their eyes to understand the world.

Strollers and Other Walkables

For strollers and bassinets, consider finding a model that can face toward you as you push it. Since they can't necessarily hear your voice, your baby may want the reassurance of seeing you to know you're still there, and it lets you continue to sign and communicate as you walk around: "Look, a fire truck!" "Wave to the doggie!"

As always, children will have their own constantly changing preferences. There came a moment when my son was done with us: he had object permanence and wanted to face forward and see the world. Luckily, we had a stroller that could switch between back and front-facing, so if you have that option, I recommend it. And if you don't have a large canopy or sunshade for when they get tuckered out, a sun blanket or other covering can be helpful to reduce visual noise.

For baby packs and carriers, the situation is reversed: worn on the front, infants will start snuggled up to you face-first. That can limit their view, so deaf kids may want to turn outward sooner than you expect. Remember, if you have a child in a front carrier facing out, you can sign in front of them and on their bodies. If your kid is in a backpack, keep in mind that they might not have a full view of your hands or face, so you might consider signing somewhat higher up on your body to give them a clear view. It also gives them the opportunity to covertly drop hearing aids or CI processors behind your back, so stay vigilant!

Car Wars

Deaf kids are more likely to be traveling long distances to special programs or for clinical visits, so there may be a lot of car time in your child's life. But car seats tend to place your child below the level of the windows and have padding that limits their sideways view of things. This means that your visual kid may end up staring at upholstery until they're old enough to potty train. This is also an issue if your child needs to see you for reassurance, or if your toddler wants to look at something other than the stains on the headrest.

Car seat mirrors are one solution: they can keep you visible to your child when you're on the road and give them a view out the front. There are many different models and ways to set them up, and some mirrors have integrated light shows or cameras that feed back to a monitor up front, among other doodads. Experiment with different arrangements; you can also add a second dedicated mirror to your dashboard or another location just for back-to-front communication so you don't have to futz with the rear-view.

Hearing Devices on the Road

They're a huge pain in the ass, actually. Depending on the device type and how they fit on your child's head, it's very easy to knock hearing aids, BAHAs, CI processors, and coils off in a stroller, carrier, or car seat. This is especially true for an infant who needs to be tilted back or stabilized with head padding. As they move their heads around, babies tend to generate screechy feedback with hearing aids, and since CI coils in particular are magnetic, they have the additional problem of sticking to any metal parts near your kid's head and pulling the coil off.

In car seats, a child will often be out of view and out of reach, so a loose HA or CI is at risk of being lost, damaged, or eaten. While there are some workarounds—wig tape, pilot caps, creative CI, or softband BAHA placement—there isn't a foolproof fix for these problems, except to take off the devices. As your child gets older and is able to sit more upright, the problem gets better, but until your child is old enough not to chew on the devices and fix these things themselves, you'll always have to be on your toes. It helps to keep a specialized case or container in the car where the devices always go; that way, you're not losing track of them in your pocket or purse, or wondering if they were left somewhere deep in the ball pit at McDonald's.

With our son, after a few weeks of futzing with his CIs constantly in the car, we settled on a system where we automatically took them off and stowed them whenever he was in a car seat. Once we got into the routine, it worked until he was about eighteen months old. Then he started asking for them back on; this created another problem when he'd get upset when they were knocked off and he couldn't fix the problem himself. This sometimes meant pulling over to fix things if it was just him and me, or sifting through stale Cheerios in the back seat looking for a dropped processor. Eventually, he got old enough and skilled enough to put his processors on and fix his coils himself if they fell off. Eventually.

Playgrounds

You should take your kid to the playground every day if you can. Kids need to move and be outside; even a not-yet-crawling baby benefits from getting out of the house and eating a little dirt. Indoor playgrounds can be a good option, too, especially in cold weather, but they are loud. Even at outdoor playgrounds, the ambient noise can get really high. So if you are speaking with your child, remember that they may not be able to understand you over the din. And if they're mobile, you won't get to object if they decide to skydive off the top of the jungle gym. Keep your eyes peeled and make sure to sit where there are some clear sight lines so you can communicate when you need to.

If your baby is really young, you'll be mostly sitting with them and watching the big kids play, but don't pass up the opportunity to sign to them, tell them what's happening, and ask questions about what they see. Watching social interactions is a major way kids learn, and if your child can't pick up the details of conversations between other people, you can fill in the gaps.

Signing in Public

The playground is a great place to practice your sign language. As a beginner, you might feel shy about using your ASL on the street, but babies and toddlers are great, non-judgmental language partners. Not only can you sign with your kid, you can sign with any little goober in the sandbox. It actually helps to reinforce language learning for your child if they see you signing to someone else, and it's adorable to watch the hearing babies all line up, hypnotized, as they try to decode this new language for themselves.

If you feel self-conscious, remember that nobody at the park actually knows ASL except you and your baby, and your baby *loves* you and *loves* it when you sign. Even if you're struggling to just say DIAPER WET?, adults will automatically assume you're some kind of hyperlinguistic brain genius.

Sooner or later, someone is going to ask, in muted awe, "How did you get fluent in ASL?"

And if you happen to run into a person who's *actually* fluent in ASL, it's going to be a Deaf parent, CODA, interpreter, or educator of some kind; I guarantee they're rooting for you and your kid, so keep it up.

Gender plays a role: in our lovely world, strangers will consider virtually anything fathers do with children, no matter how basic or half-assed, to be amazing, beyond-the-call service. Mothers, on the other hand, can expect a lot more "helpful suggestions" and other passive-aggressive judgment just for getting through the day. If you run into anyone who has unsolicited advice on raising a deaf child, make sure to get their home number. That way, when your child is awake and screaming at 2:00 a.m., you can call them over to solve any problems you might be encountering. Since they know so much.

For more pushback against bad wisdom on the playground, please refer to *Snappy Answers to Stupid Questions* in Part 5.

Hearing Devices in the Dirt

Playgrounds are great places for your child to develop their personal autonomy and physical abilities. Because of this, they're also a great place to lose hearing technology. Kids will fling off their devices doing somersaults, outrun them like Wile E. Coyote dashing off a cliff, or just pull them out for fun—or have a playmate do it for them. CIs and some BAHAs can be particularly sneaky because their magnets allow them to get stuck in weird places like the underside of a metal slide or the chain of a swing. And sand, mud, snow, and wood chips can swallow any expensive little bit of hardware without a trace.

Newer hearing devices may actually have Bluetooth tracking built in, which will tell your phone approximately where they are if you lose them. Make sure you get the tracking programs set up *before* you go out, because you can't do this once they're lost, and they can be a lifesaver. However, the trackers are generally only accurate down to about a ten-foot radius, and the signals get deflected by different materials and rely on the device battery, so you may still need to mount a major search operation.

Prevention is the name of the game. There are a variety of caps and tethers you can use to try and keep them stuck to your child—including the exclusive "bear hat" design, which you can find at willfertman.com. But if you're really worried about losing track, you can always let your kid go without devices.

Very often we arrive at a park with my son wearing his CIs, but then remove them for some especially active games, and keep them off until he asks for them back. Giving him that choice has helped him make decisions about when and how he wants to use them in other contexts, and made them very much "his," not "ours."

All-Abilities Playgrounds

If you or your child use a mobility device, are Deafblind or low vision, or have other disabilities that make typical playgrounds less than thrilling to visit, it's worth hitting Google Maps to see if there's an *all-abilities* playground nearby. While they're built to be accessible to kids and caregivers with disabilities, all-abilities playgrounds just tend to be more creative and exciting than the average swing-and-jungle-gym. The ones near our home have features like seesaws large enough to accommodate wheelchairs, Lay-Z-Boy-style swings for kids who need extra support, mazy ramp structures with slides going off in all directions that you can navigate by touch, merry-go-rounds set flush with the ground for easy access, cool sensory gardens with dozens of different-smelling herbs and flowers, and braille signage and ASL primers posted in the play areas for reference.

They're starting to crop up across the United States; the one closest to us has become our go-to for birthday parties because it can easily keep a dozen kids entertained for the requisite two hours + pizza and cupcakes. Check 'em out.

Playgroups, Finding, and Making

I'm at the playground with Oscar when I spot a boy his age with a hearing aid. Oscar doesn't have his CIs on, but I encourage him to go over and introduce himself.

He marches straight to the kid, and asks, in English,
"Do you know the language that we use when we're not wearing our hearing devices?"
It was a rocky start, but they're still friends.

The scarcity of deaf children means that you can't rely on luck to bring them together outside of school or day programs—you need to actively seek out opportunities to socialize. Families with deaf children tend to be spread out, so scheduling a day at the park makes it easier for everyone to travel to one central location. And because we're talking about parents with small children—the master saboteurs—a group playdate makes it more likely that at least a few families will actually show up; at one point, we had forty families in our playgroup, but we were lucky if five came to any one event.

Deaf playgroups may already exist in your area, but they might not be well-advertised, so scour social media and ask at your local program, school, or deaf services agency. If you can't find one, you can make a playgroup of your own. We used meetup.com to organize a local get-together, but it doesn't really matter how you do it—just remember that it's harder for folks to find you if you're using a group chat or private email chain.

Besides your deaf child, playgroups are great opportunities to expose hearing siblings to ASL and Deaf culture in a low-pressure way, but playgroups aren't only helpful for the kids: building parent-peer networks is an important survival tactic. Parenting can be lonely, and parenting a deaf child is even more isolating; having access to other hearing parents who share your experience can be a huge relief.

Playgroups are also an opportunity for you to meet and socialize with *Deaf* parents in a low-pressure environment, and give you an opportunity to meet a bigger slice of the Deaf community than you would just hanging around the deaf school or regional program. Not just families who aren't in the same programs as your kids, but also Deaf parents with hearing children, interpreters with families, and adult CODAs might also want to join to give their kids exposure to signing peers.

Both hearing and Deaf parents can be important resources for information on programs, professionals, and local opportunities for your kids; a lot of this information isn't documented anywhere but passes through word-of-mouth or the Deaf grapevine. Deaf parents are also going to have valuable perspectives on raising your children that you might not get, even from other Deaf professionals. And honestly, it's nice to hang out with folks for whom this is all just normal stuff.

If you're running your own group, especially if you're advertising to new families, setting ground rules around communication is important if you want a chance to practice your ASL and make it a good environment Deaf parents. Just remember that the more rules you set, the fewer families you'll attract, so it pays to be flexible.

Here's how we advertised ours:
> This is an ASL-based playgroup for families with Deaf, hard of hearing or CODA kids, ages infant and up. Families will meet up at different playgrounds or parks on weekends throughout the year. It's a low-key way to keep up language skills and have fun.
> 1. Drop-ins welcome.
> 2. All ASL skill levels welcome.
> 3. Bring your own snacks and water.
> 4. All kids need to have at least one parent in attendance.

In practice, that meant a spectrum of families and communication styles at the event—it's not a perfect "voices off" experience, but it set expectations pretty well, and that works for us.

Errands

Le Supermarket

The grocery store is just about the best place to bring your deaf baby from a developmental standpoint. They're brightly lit, chock-full of sensory information and easy-to-sign vocabulary, and the shopping carts make your child a captive audience.

Bring your kid to the store, show them the food. Sign the names, describe the colors, ask them if it smells good or stinky. Count the eggs. Look for animal pictures on the packaging. Fingerspell "Clabber Girl Brand Baking Powder." Just go for it! ASL 1 and 2 cover most of the food names you'll want. Show 'em a banana, sign BANANA, then feed them the banana; language learning, essential nutrition, and understated shoplifting in one convenient package.

Other Shopping

Anything you can do at the grocery store you can do at the drug store, the hardware store, the dry cleaner, or the junkyard. Remember that deaf kids often miss absorbing information secondhand, so be sure to talk about what you're buying and why you need something.

"This is medicine. I will drink it for my runny nose."

"This is a wrench. We use it to fix the sink." etc.

If you're signing, a lot of the vocabulary will be new, so having an ASL dictionary or website up on your phone is a good idea. But don't get too bogged down—if you don't know the ASL word for WRENCH, you can always fingerspell it, describe it, and use some gestures to help explain.

> *Things You Can Do with Your Kid When Your ASL Gets Good*
> - Mad Libs
> - palm reading
> - interpret the Furby
> - explain the offside rule
> - the birds and bees
> - *Rap God*
> - Pig Latin
> - define "frenemy"
> - Approach random Deaf strangers at the donut shop to figure out whom you know in common

The Beach and the Pool

Let's just stipulate that water—whether it's the ocean, a lake, river, pond, pool, waterslide, or splash park—is awesome and worth visiting as much as possible. Unfortunately, drowning is a major childhood hazard, so water is one of those things you need to take seriously.

Luckily, there's nothing innately unsafe about being a deaf swimmer. The greatest lifeguard in history, with over 900 confirmed saves, was Texas School for the Deaf graduate LeRoy Colombo. Besides regularly hauling hearing people out of Galveston riptides, he was a deep-water ocean racer, winning medals and kicking sharks into his fifties. So if Aquaman is Deaf, *your* kid will be fine in the water, but doing a little preparation is going to make the experience much safer and less stressful. As always, the key is to think visually, plan ahead, and not rely on their least reliable sense in an emergency.

Preparing for the Trip

Before you go, talk to your child about what the place will be like. Describe it as best you can, what you'll see, and what you plan on doing there. If they're mobile, discuss what your personal rules are before you arrive: stay with dad, always wear a life vest, never go deeper than your belly button. . . whatever is appropriate for your child's age, maturity, and swimming abilities. If it's a public area with rules, you may be able to find those ahead of time and talk them over with your kid too.

If your child uses hearing technology, decide together how you're going to manage it. And regardless of what kind of devices they might use, make sure you and your kid know all the signed vocabulary you'll need in an emergency: WAIT, HELP, OUT, LIFEGUARD, ICE CREAM, and so on.

Doing this ahead of time means not fighting for their attention in a new and exciting place. It gives them a chance to mentally prepare for the trip—most kids do better if they have previews of new experiences—and have at least a baseline expectation of safe behavior. It also ensures that you'll have clear lines of communication ready for when they go nuts with their cousins on the diving board. Finally, it allows you to know whether those three thousand dollar hearing aids are safe in a zip-lock bag in the car, or lost at the bottom of the Black Lagoon.

When you arrive, try to set up in a spot where you can keep in visual contact if your child heads toward the water. If there are lifeguards, you can let them know that your kid is deaf and won't necessarily hear verbal commands. Hot tip: using the word "deaf," not "hard of hearing" or "hearing loss," stops lifeguards from just trying to **yell louder** to get their attention and prompts them to use gesture and visual communication instead.

Beyond that, playground rules apply. Being at the beach or pool is multisensory in ways few other experiences are. Point out the different kinds of people around you and interpret their conversations. Describe the wildlife. Ask your kid questions about what they're experiencing. Have a splash fight, build a sand castle, eat popsicles and fried clams. Let them wander off a little and play with other children, or just dig a hole or collect shells by themselves. Free and unstructured play is important for all kids, and the water gives them unlimited opportunities to do it.

Hearing Devices in the Water

Honestly, because of the limits of hearing devices, the high cost of replacing a lost or ruined unit, and the sensory richness of the environment, beach time and pool time are particularly good moments to go technology-free.

Noise is one common factor. White noise levels on a windy beach or busy pool can be off the charts; even kids with good comprehension at home can struggle to hear you if it's breezy or echo-y.

Moisture is the biggest obstacle; there are practically no waterproof hearing aids or BAHAs on the market. Some might survive getting sprinkled or sweat on, but not dunked, especially in salt water. For the rest, the best you can do is slip on little spandex covers that will protect from splashes—check your manufacturer's recommendations.

CI users have it a little better. Most processors are water-resistant and will survive a splash, and Advanced Bionics even offers a fully waterproof processor. On top of that, there are waterproofing kits available for most models that can protect them when fully submerged, but they can be bulky and have a limited lifespan before they start to leak. Again, the manufacturer will have full details.

If a device does get wet, remove the batteries immediately and dry it with a towel, then let it dry out on its own or in a special hearing aid/CI dryer as per the manufacturer's instructions.

And if your kid gets in the water with a waterproof device, make sure you have them secured to a swim cap, swim shirt, lanyard, or some other scheme to keep them firmly attached to their body. Losing a gadget in murky or moving water can mean losing it for good. Specialized swim gear for CIs is available, which can keep the bits together a little more securely.

Other environmental hazards are direct sun, sunscreen, or sand and mud, which will cook, clog, or just devour your kid's technology. Have a safe place to stow devices: either the manufacturer's case or another sealed container. Don't do the retainer thing and wrap it in a napkin, or plunk it into unmarked Tupperware, though—that story ends with you digging through the beach dumpster along with the seagulls.

Eye and Ear Protection

Other important gear to consider for swimming are sunglasses/goggles, and ear plugs. Although not all kids like to wear them, sunglasses or swim goggles can help your visual baby see more, and feel more secure in a bright and blurry environment. Ear or nose plugs might also be important if your child has anatomical issues with drainage. Getting water into an ear that has trouble clearing it out can be painful and lead to infections. If your kid has ear tubes/grommets or other problems with their ear canal, eustachian tubes, or sinuses, talk to your doctor before you take the plunge.

Swim Lessons

If you can find them, accessible swimming lessons are precious. Swimming is a lifelong safety skill, and it opens the doors to a lot of other amazing experiences. It can be very hard to locate deaf-savvy swim instructors; check with your local deaf school and deaf services agency to start, along with local parents' groups like Hands and Voices. Remember that nearly all public and private institutions are required to accommodate your kid under the Americans with Disabilities Act at no additional cost to you (and small businesses get a tax credit for doing so), so getting an interpreter into the pool with them is a real possibility.

The Wilderness

Wild areas are another amazing place to bring your child. Deaf kids can spend a lot of time indoors or in transit, and because of the different interventions and services they get, deaf children can have more intense days than their hearing peers. And especially when our kids are young, we parents are along for the ride, having intense days of our own.

Getting some fresh air can help everyone in the family decompress, whether that's a hike up a mountain, fishing off a pier, or a cookout at the park. Nature will meet your baby on equal terms—there's an infinite array of things to see, smell, touch, climb, and explore, and there's no wrong way to play with a stick.

Deaf culture has a lot of appreciation for the wilderness, and you can find plenty of Deaf hiking groups and outdoor enthusiasts, so it's worth checking to see if there are organizations or meetups in your neighborhood. State and national parks will often also have interpreted tours or signing park rangers you can connect with, too. (And check out the National Parks Access Pass below!)

Preparing for the Trip

Like the beach, it's a good idea to give a preview before you leave, when you have your child's attention. Describe where you're going, and what you'll see and do when you get there. Preparing kids for outings in this way can make it a lot more fun for both of you—they'll arrive excited and primed to look for bluejays or mushrooms, and you can set expectations for their behavior and lock down critical sign vocabulary.

If you're going farther than the park, be very explicit about safety rules. Just remember that there's a line between preparing kids and freaking them out, especially for young children. Keep explanations direct and matter-of-fact:

"If you see a snake, don't get close or touch it. It doesn't like people."

"Don't walk through plants on the sides of the trail. Some of them are poison oak, and they can make you itchy."

If your child uses hearing technology, figuring out the battery situation before you leave will also be important, especially if you're staying overnight where there isn't an easy way to charge or replace batteries. Hiking back to the car after dark to retrieve the backups is nobody's idea of fun.

Making a plan for getting lost or separated on a walk is especially important for more mobile kids who can run ahead, fall behind, or just get distracted at the wrong moment. They should know to wait for the group if they come to a fork in the path, stick to the middle of the trail, and stay put if they're lost and not hide from adults who might be able to help.

Although a lot of outdoor gear tends to come in earth tones, try to wear bright colors if you're out in the woods—it will help you stay in visual contact. Flashlights are important for the same reason, so make sure everyone's got one if you're camping or hiking near sunset. Bring lanterns and spare batteries for the campsite, too; light equals communication! Finally, if your child is mobile enough to get lost on their own, they should also have your contact info somewhere on their person, along with information about communicating with them.

Ultimately, though, taking kids into nature means allowing them to run ahead and letting them get a little scratched up. Calculated danger is the goal here. Kids who take small risks reap big rewards in terms of independence.

Orienteering

If you're going for a hike, grab any maps that are available, and show your kid the route, along with trail markers and signs as you go. Point out cardinal directions and teach them how to use a compass if you've got one handy. Because of their visual powers, deaf kids can develop excellent orientation skills, and teaching them how to read a map and navigate is going to be a valuable lifelong skill.

Tracking Devices

One nice thing about hearing technology these days: in a true emergency, if you have cell reception, the tracking features on some hearing aids and CI processors can also help you locate your child. But that's a big if; the devices have to be switched on, they have to be with your kid, and you need to be close to a cell tower. So make sure you've got less technical strategies in place, too.

National Park Access Pass

This is one of the best deals in the universe: the US government offers free lifetime entry to the families of deaf children at over 2000 national parks and recreation areas all over the country. It's called the "Access Pass," and it's available for US citizens or permanent residents of any age who have a "permanent disability," which includes deafness. You can obtain it for your baby, and it will admit them plus any three adults riding in the same car into a national park for free (siblings under sixteen get in for free in any case). Google it!

Snow and Cold

Snow is awesome. Playing in snow, building snow people, having snowball fights, sledding, skiing, skating . . . if you've got snow you've got fun. On the other hand, cold is a fact of life. If you live in a cold climate, you've got to deal with it.

Keeping Your Hands Warm for Signing

If you live somewhere with real winters, finding ways to keep your hands warm and visible is important. You need to protect your fingers, but stiff conventional gloves might make it difficult to both sign and be understood. For chilly weather, consider lightweight stretch gloves or glove liners. Make sure the color is high-contrast so you're not signing with black gloves against a black jacket, or white gloves against the snow!

If you need to be warmer, you can also use mittens and just pull them off to sign and then slip them back on. Clips that keep them attached to the sleeves will make this easier for the kids. Another option is fingerless hunter's gloves, where the mitten part flips up from the back. No matter what you decide for yourself and your child, test it out to make sure you can both understand each other.

Eye and Ear Protection

Snowy weather is another situation where goggles or sunglasses might be important for a visual kid. Both blowing snow and glare from sunlight in the wintertime can make it hard to see and communicate. Of course, on a ski or snowboard trip, or anywhere you'll be out in the glare all day, you need to protect your child's eyes from UV light with quality polarized goggles.

When you bundle up your kid, keep in mind the way different hats, scarves, and high collars on snow jackets can block your child's vision; you may have to experiment to find combinations of snow clothes that give your kid the widest field of view. If your child uses hearing devices, make sure the microphones are not scraping against a hat or other clothing; that'll just annoy them and keep them from hearing anything. Depending on the particular device, they can be secured under hats or earmuffs if they don't move around. Note that a CI's magnetic coils work fine through cloth, so you can always stick them on the outside of a lightweight cap if needed.

Hearing Devices in the Snow

First of all, never put cold devices onto or into your kid's ears! If your child's doodads have been hanging around outside, warm them up in your hands or in a pocket first.

Cold weather is hard on hearing technology. Batteries will run down fast, so bring spares, and avoid leaving them outside or in a cold car. Rapid temperature changes can cause moisture to condense inside devices, which can easily damage them. For HAs, those water-resistant spandex covers will give a bit of extra protection from condensation externally, but not for the internals. For CIs, you can potentially put them into a water protection kit if they're likely to get wet, but that also won't help with internal condensation. Be prepared to pull the batteries and pop them into a drying kit when you're done, even if they seem dry. You really want to clear up any water that ends up in the tubes or circuits.

Wearing hearing devices day-to-day in the cold shouldn't be an issue. But when considering snow play, deaf kids are just a lot more durable than their electronics. Between hats, wet weather, temperature stress, battery life, and the possibility of losing something in a snow bank until the spring thaw, leaving gadgets at home or in a warm pocket might be the better option if you plan to have some serious winter fun.

Museums, Concerts, and Events

If you're like our family, free stuff in the park is a major part of the weekend. We're lucky to live in an area where a performance or fair is always happening, and we're usually there with a blanket and a frisbee. Parents sometimes worry about bringing deaf kids to "hearing" events like concerts for fear that they'll feel left out or not get anything out of them. Access *is* important: keeping an eye out for accessible or Deaf cultural events is part of your job description, as is calling ahead to secure interpreters or other access for your child. But it's also important to expose your kid to all the things and not pre-judge what they'll enjoy or if they're enjoying it "the right way."

Keep an eye on them when doing something new, and debrief them after an event to make sure they felt included, if not entertained. A little *strategic* boredom is a great parenting tool and builds, um, "character." But endless, tedious exclusion is the dull knife of dinner table syndrome and will guarantee your future placement in a miserable nursing home.

For many events, hearing levels just aren't an issue. The rides at the county fair don't care: the Gravitron just wants to make you barf.[6] Even for more sound-centric events, you can bring some toys and books or other kid gear to hedge your bet.

Last year, we took the boys to the Hardly Strictly Bluegrass Festival in Golden Gate Park. It's a massive free concert in downtown San Francisco with multiple stages. Oscar decided he didn't want to wear his CIs for the show, but he had a blast anyhow, playing in the grass with his brother, watching the people and the performers, and enjoying the sensations from the giant sound system while we picnicked.

On the other hand, museums and other venues will sometimes have free or low-cost tickets and ASL-interpreted events for deaf children and their families. Stick to social media and you'll find a lot, and don't be shy about contacting the box office or front desk to ask what they have to offer; big organizations will have ADA coordinators or offices that handle this.

---

[6]But put those hearing aids / CIs in a pocket before you get on the rides!!!

Even if you're paying full price, accessible shows and tours shouldn't cost extra, although often only one or two time slots will be offered. You sometimes have to guarantee a certain number of tickets before they'll hire the terp, so you've got to be flexible with the schedule and network with other parents. Our local children's theater always has interpreted performances, and their *Frog and Toad* kicked ass. We sat in the reserved Deaf seating near the front with a bunch of Oscar's buddies and got a double show from both the actors on stage and the theatrical interpreters down front. For more tips on events, see *Interpreters, Hiring and Firing*.

For truly loud stuff like indoor concerts, sports events, or monster truck rallies, you'll want to ask your kid's audiologist about protecting their residual hearing. Depending on your situation, they may recommend headphones or other precautions. But besides that, go nuts.

Reading to Your Deaf Child

Night.

Bathtime is over. Oscar is lying on the rug in his bedroom, wrapped in a towel. His CIs are off, and he's ready for stories. He's rejected all the easy books, so I'm cross-legged on the floor, making shaky progress on Alligator Baby in my crappy ASL.

Halfway through, Oscar turns his head away, and closes his eyes.
He pulls the towel over his face. His breathing is steady. All is quiet.
A minute passes. I stop signing.

From under the towel, a roar: **"Keep reading!"**

Books are a vital part of raising a deaf baby. You should read to your child every day, in whatever ways you can. I don't need to give you the usual "literacy is important" speech, but beyond the obvious reasons—work, school, *Dog Man*—reading is a key aspect of getting your kid ready for life as a deaf person. The written word is one of the essential ways deaf adults access the hearing world: closed captions, CART, note takers in school, texting or emailing rather than calling, writing your Starbucks order on a sticky note, and so on. Do not miss this boat.

The Literacy Boogeyman

Be warned—if you've got a deaf child, one of the ghost stories you'll encounter from bad educators will go like this:

- Your child needs to learn to read and write English.
- ASL is not English, and has no written form.

Therefore…

- Your child has got to listen and speak.
- Your child must get a CI.
- Your child must use Signed Exact English or Cued Speech.
- Your child must mainstream with hearing kids.

    etc.

This line of thinking has cursed deaf children with language deprivation and poor literacy skills for more than a century.

The truth is, like a lot of languages around the world, ASL does *not* have an official written form. There are ways of depicting ASL on the page, like gloss or signwriting, but typically, when Deaf folks want to write something down, even for other Deaf people, they write in English. This might seem weird, because in the United States we generally grow up learning to read and write the same language that we speak, but it's actually a common situation worldwide. In places like China and the Arab world, tens of millions of hearing people speak a home language that's very different from the Mandarin Chinese or classical Arabic they read and write in school.

In the Deaf world, it's routine for Deaf parents to raise literate bilingual Deaf kids who never get within a hundred miles of an "oral education." Deaf-of-Deaf children typically have English reading and writing skills on par with their hearing peers, even if they've never spoken a word. Studies of Deaf families explain why: early access to ASL prevents language deprivation and builds basic linguistic competence. Once a child's brain has a strong basis in one language, they can easily transfer those skills to a second or third language.

This doesn't mean that every Deaf person is a great reader or eloquent writer, although some certainly are. Plenty of Deaf adults were subject to the inadequate and abusive educational bullshit you're trying to avoid for your child, and this left parts of the community without strong English skills. But even this fact tends to get thrown at hearing parents: "Those terrible Deafs can't even spell right!"

Don't believe it for a second.

Reading to Your Baby

To raise a strong reader, you don't need hearing devices, signed English, or spoken language at all, but you do need to expose your child to books and to reading from the very beginning. That means getting children's books into the house—a library card helps—and setting aside time to read to your child every day, for at least twenty or thirty minutes.

Depending on where your child's hearing is at and what their preferences are, you may be reading to them exclusively in ASL, or sometimes in ASL, and sometimes in spoken English, or in whatever languages your family uses at home.

Reading to a young baby can feel silly, especially a deaf baby, but keep going. They will appreciate being snuggled, having you close, and communicating with them, even if they've got no idea what you're saying. As they get deeper into their babyhood, they'll start learning that the colorful rectangle in front of them has meaning in it, and that it feels good to chew when they're teething. The books will get torn the hell up, and that's ok—just lay in a lot of tape for repairs. Sooner or later, they will connect the idea of pictures and then letters and words to the story.

Reading in ASL

Even if you're just starting to learn, there are a lot of benefits to signing books for you and your child. Not only does it give your baby a chance to start making those early connections between books and language, but it's a perfect way for you to practice your ASL. After all, kids' books are designed to support language. Their simple, repetitive stories, with picture cues and basic vocabulary, will help you practice your signs, learn important phrases, and build up your confidence. And babies demand repetition, so you'll have a dozen memorized in no time!

When you first start, you will need to preview stories, look up different words, think about classifiers, and consult with teachers or mentors to figure out how to say things correctly in ASL. It's more work than just grabbing something off the shelf, but figuring out an interpretation and then signing it to your kid feels like a real accomplishment, and each book added to the pile will build your confidence. Because Oscar was identified as deaf very early, we began to read to him in our beginner's ASL from when he was about three months old. Now that he's five, I'm still not a super-confident signer, but I can crank out a slick version of *Brown Bear, Brown Bear, What Do You See?* on demand.

Don't worry if your ASL isn't "good enough"—your baby is the most forgiving audience you could imagine. Just do your best, and they will love the time you take to pay attention to them and communicate. Kids are extraordinary linguists, and if they're being exposed to fluent ASL elsewhere, they'll filter out mistakes you might make and just pick up the right stuff. You can actually see this process in immigrant families. Parents who come to the United States from other countries may not be native speakers, but their children understand mom and dad's English just fine. Not only that, but they grow up to speak the local American dialect flawlessly. Baby brains are powerful!

Setting Up for ASL Reading Time

You'll quickly notice something different about reading in sign language, and it's a clue to a lot of other differences in your kid's development. Compared to passively listening, vision is an active sense. While a hearing child might sit in your lap and look only at the book while the story is read, your deaf kid needs to watch your face, hands, and the book, all at once, and move their eyes from one to another to keep up with the story. This kind of strong *joint visual attention* and *gaze shifting* are key abilities for deaf children, and it's one reason why deaf kids aren't just "kids who can't hear"—they have a different experience of the world and develop different skills for dealing with it.

There are two ways you can handle positioning when reading in sign language: face your kid and sign toward them, or sit them in your lap facing away and sign on their body. Having them sit on your lap is nice because it's cozy for them and comfortable for you. It lets kids reach out and touch the book and turn pages, and it supports phonological awareness when you place a sign in the correct place on their body (or place *their* hands in the correct place). But it's also limited because they may not be able to see your expression, and unless it's a very simple book, or you're a very skillful signer, you won't always be able to put across the story from behind them. Sitting in front of a large mirror (like a closet mirror) can help, letting your child gaze-shift between you and the book.

Signing while facing your child has a different challenge; you need to prop up both the book AND your baby. This can require some creative arrangements, especially before your kid can sit / stand on their own. High chairs and bouncy seats are great for this (so books can be a mealtime thing), or sitting them on your bed with pillows can work, too. For us, once he could stand with support, Oscar's best reading spot was his crib: he'd stand holding the rails while I faced him and signed sitting in a chair.

You might also need to have a place to put your book so it stays open while you sign with both hands. Sometimes you can just unfold it in your lap or go at it one-handed, but a rubber band, hair tie, book weight, hair clip, chip clip, music stand, or recipe / cookbook stand can work, too. I personally kept some extra board books around that I could use to prop the one I was reading open. This can also limit your kid's ability to interact with the book, so make sure you let them examine and play with it, too.

I'm a firm believer that physical books are better for kids, but if you have difficulty with positioning or securing a book, or if it's easier to borrow books digitally, you can set up a storybook as a slideshow on a laptop, tablet, or phone that leaves both your hands free. Just don't neglect the power of a paper book as a learning tool—kids learn with their hands (and mouths!) as well as their eyes, and need to be able to explore books independently as well as in your lap.

Finding Books to Sign

To start, grab some very simple baby books—the kind without any plot. Board books that are basically lists of emotions, colors, animals, opposites, the alphabet, and so on, are everywhere. "First 100 word" books are great because they focus on kid-specific vocabulary, so you can learn the basics along with your child. The best part is that you can point to the picture and sign a single word without needing to get into the nitty-gritty of ASL grammar.

Next steps can be repetitive story or concept books like Martin and Carle's *Brown Bear, Brown Bear* or Patricelli's *Baby Happy, Baby Sad*. You just need to master the key phrase and then swap out one or two words. Wordless or near-wordless books like *Good Dog, Carl* are also wonderful to start with, because they allow you to only describe as much as you can; as your sign becomes stronger, you'll be able to tell more of the story.

As time goes on, you'll be able to expand your selection. You'll find some books naturally lend themselves to ASL; *Everyone Poops* is fun, and so is *Go Dog Go*, but others are going to be difficult no matter how good you get. Stories that rely on English-language rhymes can be tough to make "work" in ASL; Dr. Seuss is the mountain we all must eventually climb.[7] But even if you find yourself struggling with the vocabulary in a particular book, you can always downshift and just look at the pictures and discuss them together, or use the next strategy:

Interactive Reading and Conceptual Translation

When reading to your child, don't just plow through the story if you can help it. Stop and ask them questions about what they see, point out your favorite parts, or even get a part "wrong" and see if your baby notices. You will be signing these same books hundreds of times, and as your skills improve, there will be more opportunities for you to play, and playing is always right.

As your child grows older, more complex books will also require you to interpret the book more aggressively. Just like translating between any two languages, a straightforward word-for-word rendering might not make much sense.

---

[7]If you really want to nerd out and see just how incredible an ASL interpretation can be, find some Crom Saunders interpretations of Shel Silverstein, or Joe Valez's *Jabberwoky*, possibly the greatest piece of ASL theater ever made.

> It's hard to describe to a native speaker just how inexplicable English can be, and it's big obstacle teaching literacy to Deaf children. For example, 'once upon a time.' What the hell does that mean? Or 'put out the fire'—you take the fire outside?
>
> Parents can help their children a lot by aiming straight for the meaning of a phrase or sentence, instead of focusing on individual words.
>
> Rachel Zemach, Deaf author and educator

This process is called *conceptual translation*; you tell the story of what happens in the book instead of repeating every word written down on the page. It can be tricky at first; the urge to follow the text exactly can be strong, but as you practice a particular book, you'll develop your own way of reading a story and become more skillful in expressing your version.

Don't worry about your reading not being "the real story" or "real English." Studies show that Deaf parents, who are hands-down the best at teaching Deaf children to read, typically start reading a new book with a conceptual translation, and then home in on specific words or phrases and demonstrate the relationship between ASL and English. Children can then build a bridge between the two languages: you can show them that "once upon a time" in English means "a long time ago" in ASL, or that to "put out" a fire really means "pour water" on it. This is an advanced technique, but you will have years and plenty of help to figure it out.

Be warned that your kid's language development will eventually outpace your sign language skills—which is great! When you get to the point where your child is demanding harder books than you can manage, teachers and mentors can help pick up the slack; if you keep working on your sign, you'll catch up. In the meantime, just keep looking for new books or stories that match your child's interests, if not their language level. There are a LOT of early readers out there with simple vocabulary for kindergarteners that make great mid-level books for you to share with your child. And once you're at that level, you can always ask your child to sign a book to *you*.

Reading Aloud

If your child has access to spoken language through hearing devices, you should also read to them in English or any other languages you speak at home. And even if your child has very low levels of hearing and you're not yet confident with your ASL, you can still read to them with a lot of gestures, expressions, miming, and pointing! Just getting the message across that the book has fun information inside it is the first step to getting your child interested in reading.

When reading aloud, try and find as quiet a space as possible, away from noise like running dishwashers or the radio, and make sure you're oriented so your kid has the best access to your voice; for instance, speaking into their preferred ear or having them snuggled to your chest so they can pick up vibrations from your body. Be aware that you might need to face your baby so they can take in visual cues from your face and the book as well as your voice, but that snuggle time is another important part of story time, so you should mix it up.

Obviously, you'll be able to tackle more complex stories in your native language at first. In our house, once our son got his CIs, I started dividing the book piles into signing and speaking books, and to this day, I keep track of which ones I'm confident signing and which I really need to read in English.

But even if your child has strong access to spoken language, you will find many moments when a signed book is what does the trick. Tired kids often take their HAs and CIs off. Or they demand books in the bathtub. Or in the middle of the night. Or when the batteries in their hearing devices are dead. Or a million other things. Get those hands up!

ASL Children's Books and Media

There are a small number of ASL-specific books and series out there that actually integrate sign into their stories in various ways: *Monster Hands* by Karen Kane and Jonaz McMillan, the *Love and Language* books by Laura Blum, the *Nita* books by Kathy MacMillan, the *Moses* series by Isaac Millman, and the *Handtalk* series by Mary Beth Miller and Remy Charlip, which also features some amazing photography by George Acona and a rad early 1980s PBS vibe.

As always, be careful of "baby sign" books that teach invented or wrong signs, or books that use other sign languages like BSL or Auslan (unless that's what you're looking for). There's also a cottage industry of parent-authored books showing kids with CIs or hearing aids out there, of varying quality. Deaf authors and authors who work closely with the Deaf community are always best.

Monster Hands, as well as the *Moses* and *Handtalk* series, are important because they explicitly feature Deaf characters in their stories. Another wonderful recent book in that vein is *Proud to be Deaf* by Lilli Beese. Although the book is about life in the UK, and so incorporates BSL, it's written from the point of view of a ten-year-old Deaf girl, and it's fabulous for giving your kid some role models in print and really instilling some Deaf pride.

For more of my favorite books for deaf kids, go to willfertman.com.

ASL Children's Book Videos

We are living in a golden age of signed books: YouTube is the gift that keeps giving, and there are a lot of great children's books available now in ASL interpretations from Deaf educators. They're perfect for watching with your kid and reviewing yourself for your own practice. Many deaf schools put out these videos; Rocky Mountain Deaf School and Texas Statewide Outreach Center, in particular put out a lot of great stories on YouTube, with strong production values and skillful signers. But remember that however good a video is, they're no substitute for *you* reading books with your child. No matter how insecure you feel about your signing, sitting there and communicating with your baby in person is worth a million hours of RMDSCO.

For reading along with your child, there's also Motion Light Lab's VL2 storysigning books for iPad, which are children's books with integrated ASL in them, so you can switch back and forth between written text and signing at any point in the story. These are great for emerging readers as texts that bridge ASL and English.

ASL Storytelling, Rhythms and Rhymes, and Other Fun Stuff

Besides interpretations of kids' books, Deaf culture has native story traditions you need to know about. Storytelling is an art that's been around ever since Deaf people have shared language, and storytelling skills are highly valued in Deaf communities. There are many Deaf storytellers out there putting together videos for kids, as well as doing live shows and events.

Kid's stories can be interpretations of well-known tales like the Three Little Pigs, or they might be famous only in the Deaf community, like the Lumberjack Story, or original creations altogether. Like you'd expect from a visual culture, Deaf storytelling is vivid and dynamic, and besides regular stories, there are many unique forms that could only exist in ASL:

ABC stories are a kind of poetry made from twenty-six signs that use handshapes of the alphabet in order, from A to Z, to tell the story.

Handshape stories are almost the opposite: they tell a complete tale using only signs that have the *same* handshape.

Personification stories take on the perspective of an object or animal, like an egg on its journey from under the chicken, through the grocery store, and into a frying pan.

Visual vernacular (VV) stories are told mostly with classifiers, gesture, and mime, not signing per se, and are known for being cinematic and action-oriented, with changing "camera angles," slow motion, and other tricky techniques.

The list goes on—Deaf culture is bursting with creativity.

Rhythms and rhymes are an important form of storytelling for new parents. These are native ASL nursery rhymes that use all the usual tricks—repetition, visual rhyme, call-and-response, and so on—to amuse deaf babies. Like English nursery rhymes, they can be upbeat song-games, mini-lessons about colors or days of the week, or just sweet little lullabies. They make great fill-ins when you're waiting for an appointment, or if you want to keep your kid happy in the bathtub. And unlike a half-hour, five-man visual vernacular reenactment of *The Matrix*, they are simple: you can master a rhyme in a few minutes and use it with your child at bedtime.

Knowing a rhyme and signing it to your baby is just the beginning—they're a fun way to *play* with language with your child. As with a book, once they're familiar with a rhyme, you can have them sign along, pause the rhyme and wait for your child to fill in the next word, or deliberately get a word wrong and have your baby correct you. You can slow it down, speed it up, sign the words on their body, have them sign the words on your body, and a million other things—it's like rocket fuel for language acquisition. *Hands Land* on Amazon Prime is a great resource for rhythms and rhymes. It's written and performed by a team of Deaf language experts and has several seasons of amazing content about animals, feelings, shapes, and more. Definitely worth checking out.

Other ASL Media for Deaf Kids

There are a few other YouTube channels, websites, TV shows, and movies for deaf kids that deserve mention.

ASL Nook is a series on YouTube made by Deaf mom Sheena McFeely and her family where they teach ASL vocabulary, meet Deaf creators, and go on adventures. It's great not only for learning the language but also for seeing ordinary interactions between Deaf parents and children. They have since gone on to other things (Shaylee's in movies now!), but their videos remain.

Atomic Hands hosts science videos in ASL, featuring Deaf scientists and educators, with topics ranging from the origin of zero to the secret life of ants. Their website is ASL STEM central, with tons of resources for budding researchers.

PBS Kids has ASL-interpreted episodes of *Arthur*, *Daniel Tiger's Neighborhood*, and more, with skilled interpreters overlaid on the video. It's a beautiful day in the neighborhood.

MyGo! Sign Language for Kids has a similar series of interpreted toddler-friendly edutainment shows like *Cocomelon* and *Blippi*, so you can get your Baby Shark on.

SignUp ASL Captioning has begun doing picture-in-picture ASL captioning for popular kids' movies and television, using a plug-in for the Chrome browser that can overlay Disney+ and Netflix shows. They are adding new captioned films to their roster all the time, including absolute bangers like *Frozen* and *The Magic School Bus*.

I have more ASL storytellers, shows, and interpreted media at willfertman.com.

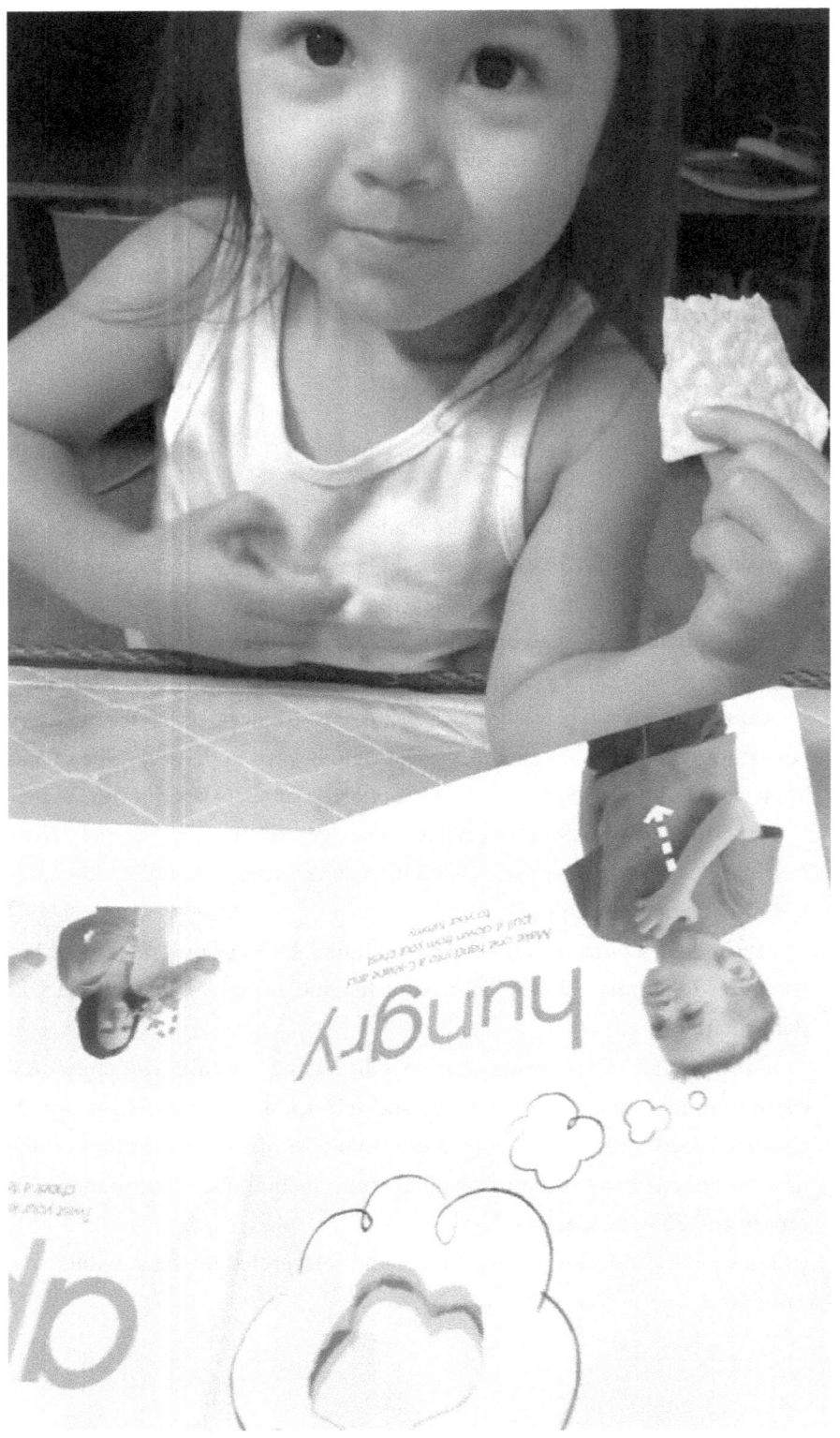

Stephanie Lucero, 2025

3

Family

"Hi, Mom. So . . . the doctors think Oscar might be deaf. They wanted to know if anyone in our family is deaf, but I can't think of anyone."

"Nobody on our side of the family is deaf.

"Except for my cousin Joy.

"And her son.

"And your great-aunt, who you're named after."

"Oh . . . Okay. How come I didn't know that?"

"Oh, you met Joy before. Don't you remember? She was at your second birthday party!"

". . ."

Dinner Table Syndrome: Not as Delicious as it Sounds

Why are we doing all this? What's the point of grinding away at ASL and strategizing about communication with your kid day-to-day? Who cares if they don't know about the trip to the hardware store or their older brother's math test? As long as they understand their teachers, what's the problem? Don't we leave our *hearing* kids out of most of our adult conversations?

Yes and no. Kids get left out of a lot of grown-up talk. It's inevitable—we protect them from upsetting or confusing stuff, and sometimes we just don't feel like answering a million "why?" questions when going over the terms of the new mortgage. But for children, growing up means watching adults and scouring them for clues about how to be in the world. As they observe, they also experiment with participating, jumping into conversations, adding their own thoughts and sharing their experiences, learning how to initiate and sustain communication. This helps them learn many of their social skills and is one of the key ways that children solicit love, attention, and praise. Just like language acquisition, a huge amount of real-world learning and relationship-building in a family isn't intentional; it's what happens when you're shooting the breeze.

"Dinner table syndrome" is the actual-factual name for the loss of incidental learning and affection that occurs when deaf children can't participate in family life.[1] It gets its name from the common scenario of a deaf kid sitting at the dinner table, isolated, while the family has a conversation around them. Someone tells a joke, and everyone else laughs. The kid asks, "What's so funny?" and the parents say, "I'll tell you later."

Here's a hint: nobody *ever* tells you later.

After language deprivation, dinner table syndrome is the most serious obstacle you will face with your deaf child. Being alone in a crowd is an awful thing, and if the crowd is your family, it can be utterly devastating. Dinner table syndrome alienates deaf kids from their parents and siblings, has a terrible impact on their mental health, and it can leave deaf adults with huge gaps in their knowledge of the world and their ability to manage relationships with others.

The sadness and rage that dinner table syndrome provokes in us Deaf people is huge. This is my family, yet I'm ninety-five percent left out, and no one even seems to be aware of it! Being alone in a bubble, while the people you love chat obliviously around you, is a painfully lonely experience. It

---

[1] Dinner table syndrome is also known as linguistic neglect, although that term can also encompass language deprivation syndrome.

causes individual, and a collective, cultural trauma—and it is common! I felt it as a pre-teen, I felt it as a young adult, and I felt it last week.

Rachel Zemach, Deaf author and educator

There's no single way to avoid dinner table syndrome—just strategies. It's a process of continually making sure your child is included in the life of your family.

Sign It

If your child needs ASL to understand you, then you need to sign when they're around. And if your child has access to spoken language but isn't using their technology or is in a situation where it doesn't work well, you need to sign then, too.

This applies not just when you are talking to your baby, but also when you are talking near your baby to other family members. Whatever the topic, use ASL if you can. Planning a trip to the DMV? Sign it. Making a shopping list? Sign it. Talking about the news? Sign it.

I don't want to be glib. For a family, going bilingual is not a fast or easy process. Setting aside your home language, even for a few minutes, can be really stressful. You're sitting down to supper after a long day, and you want to relax, but suddenly easy interactions become precarious. Details get blurry. Attention shifting is tiring, fingerspelling is tedious, and it sometimes feels silly to be doing this on behalf of the baby when everyone else in the room is hearing.

You will need to practice, have patience, and be gentle on yourself and your hearing family members. As you go along, different people are going to have different feelings and progress at different rates. Setting realistic goals for your fluency is very important as you make your way; it's the only way you're going to succeed. Just remember that making an effort to include your child prevents them from feeling that same kind of uncertainty, stress, and confusion *all the time*.

In our house, breakfast is the prime moment for signing. My deaf son doesn't like to put on his CIs first thing in the morning, so we're feeding and prepping him and his hearing brother for school in ASL, and trying to handle all the morning business in sign. Are we successful? On a good day, we make it maybe seventy-five percent in sign. On a bad day, we're maybe doing only twenty-five percent, talking around and over my son, and only using ASL when we're speaking to him directly.

This is for a lot of reasons: we'll be tired, or rushed, or my wife and I will run into a topic we don't have the vocabulary for. Our hearing kid might not have that much enthusiasm for the deaf project that morning and ignore us, or just speak his answers back to us. The ultimate passive-aggressive move is for Leo to ask us to interpret things he knows how to sign to Oscar. Our deaf kid might be feeling bratty and just scream at everything, or just wrap himself in a blanket and block out the world.

What I'm saying is, you don't need to be perfect, but you need to be persistent. Forgive yourself when you fall back on old habits, but don't give up. Remember that it's not just sharing information—communication is love.

Say It

If your child also has access to spoken language, including them in family talk can also mean changing the habits you have around spoken conversations. Even deaf kids with strong 1-on-1 English comprehension won't have the same capacity to sort out single voices in a noisy room, or necessarily follow a conversation if there are many people talking over each other.

Part of this is making sure the environment is as friendly as possible—turn off the TV, radio, dishwasher, washing machine, or anything else that might make a lot of background noise. Kitchens, in particular, tend to have the most running gadgets and a lot of hard, echo-y surfaces. Arranging your space is also important: our actual kitchen table is small and cramped, so if we want to keep our sight lines clear, we'll take our meals in the dining room.

And if you're like us and have a lot of fast, noisy, interrupt-y conversations together, you may need to slow the pace a little. Encourage turn-taking with the kids, try to keep side conversations to a minimum, and check in with your deaf child to make sure they're getting what everyone is saying. If it's too hard for your kid to follow, switch to ASL.

These habits apply to your deaf kid, too. Deaf children with access to speech can sometimes end up dominating spoken conversations; they want to participate, but will lose the thread of discussions if they don't know the topic. So they'll interrupt or bulldoze you or their siblings so that they can continue talking about subjects they're familiar with.

In our house, it can be more extreme than that: our deaf son is delighted to talk at us with his CIs off and have us sign back. This is fine if it's one-on-one, where we can easily take turns, but if he wants to talk with the whole family, we generally insist on him either switching to ASL or putting on his CIs—it's just about the only time we insist on it—because otherwise he just keeps blabbing over us with no regard for us or his poor brother, trying to get a word in edgewise.

And remember that if your deaf child is doing this sort of thing, it can indicate they're not getting enough information or context to participate—you may need to break out the sign language and employ the next major anti-dinner table tactic:

TMI

Infodumps are another strategy to prevent dinner table syndrome. Take time out to explain certain things explicitly that your child might not pick up from eavesdropping. What's life insurance? How do you tie a necktie? Where is the White House and who lives there? This isn't just for raising a good *Jeopardy!* contestant, it extends to the relationships and events in your life: What does "uncle" mean? Who's a relative and who's just a friend of the family? What do you do for work, and what is your boss's name? Make those links for your child and don't assume they'll just soak it up as you go along.

This approach can sometimes mean pausing a discussion to clarify who or what you're talking about, or pulling a kid aside to give them a rundown on a topic. It can change the flow of conversations in your family when you do this, but it's important.

You'll see this a lot in Deaf culture; Deaf adults often take extra time to explain context and define terms when they're having a conversation and are quick to ask questions if they don't understand something. Meet a Deaf person for the first time, and you're going to learn a lot more about their extended family, education, employment, and medical history than you might from a hearing person. Because knowledge was often withheld from deaf children growing up, Deaf adults don't take it for granted. The culture values sharing information, asking questions, and making sure everyone can understand and participate.

From a hearing perspective, this can sometimes seem like overkill, or the dreaded Too Much Information.[2] But keep at it and don't be embarrassed; it's going to help you raise an independent, resourceful, and loved kid.

Terp It

If your child relies on ASL, either full-time or in noisy environments, getting interpreters for appointments and events in the hearing world is going to be an important aspect of preventing dinner table syndrome as well.

An interpreter isn't just a channel of communication between your kid and their dentist. An interpreter should be signing *all* spoken conversations that happens during an appointment or event, whether it's directed at your child or not. This allows your kid to spy on the adult world the way hearing children do. It exposes them to vocabulary and concepts from different fields (medical, technical, the arts, etc.) to help round out their life experience. And skillful interpreters can also do a lot to clarify concepts for young children, so your kid will potentially understand *more* of what's happening to them than a hearing child might.

There's no lower age limit for interpreters; you can and should book them for infants. After all, hearing babies get access to language at that age, and your deaf baby's needs are no different. One positive side effect I've noticed: my kid hates medical appointments, but he's much more calm when there's an interpreter present. Having someone that's just "for him" helps him feel supported in scary places like a doctor's office.

Always having interpreters also helps prevent one of the most insidious symptoms of dinner table syndrome: the feeling that there are secret decisions

---

[2]For a spectacular example of this, watch the Daily Moth online. What would be a 30-second interview on a hearing news show turn into a 10-minute expose: watching a Deaf-run news show will get you *informed*.

being made about you behind your back. Many deaf adults have a terrible relationship with doctors, schools, landlords, and authorities and institutions of all kinds. Growing up, they were never able to monitor or participate in the choices that were being made for them, their lives, and their bodies. Being "dinner tabled" can subject you to a lot of nasty surprises, including unannounced medical procedures, inexplicable school transfers, cryptic bureaucratic appointments, and unexpected funerals.

> One day when I was 12, I came home from school and Dad said I suddenly had to be somewhere... What? Where are we going?
>
> We enter an office, sit in the waiting room, and next thing you know an old man is shoving a needle into my gums and doing all kinds of cavity-filling stuff, and that was my first dental appointment. I had TWO cavities in my mouth on my left side, one on the top and one on the bottom.
>
> Cue going home; time to eat dinner. Mom and Dad chat about my dental appointment which I don't follow at all; can't hear them. I have to chew delicately and use my right side teeth to chew which is... Different...
>
> Then Mom announced that we were having ice cream for dessert. "Who wants ice cream???"
>
> "Meeee!" "I do!" "Me, please!" Even Dad chimed in...
>
> So all of us have ice cream and I completely forgot about my cavity fillings that were done less than 2 hours prior. I chomp down on the ice cream on my left side of my mouth and immmmmmediately regret it tremendously.
>
> I was in super pain and of course Mom laughs and said, "HAHA! Now I guess you'll brush your teeth more!"
>
> Carrie, Deaf adult

A constant drip of scary and painful events, without knowing why they're happening or having any ability to change things, can leave deaf folks feeling discouraged or helpless when advocating for themselves. This is the opposite of what your kid needs—to get by in the hearing world, deaf people need *more* agency, *more* gumption, and *more* self-determination than the average. Keeping them in the loop with interpreters is part of giving them these skills.

The good news is that the ADA requires that almost all public and private facilities book interpreters at no cost to you. See the chapter *Interpreters, Hiring and Firing* later on in the book for more.

Mic It

If your child uses an FM or Bluetooth system for their hearing devices, you can bring it along for appointments as well, and make sure the doctor / teacher / whoever uses it. All the reasons I just listed for needing an interpreter apply if your child relies on HAs or CIs. Access is king, and there's no "too young."

Siblings

Me: What would you say to a family that has deaf and hearing kids?
Oscar: You should tell them that they don't need to have a real brother, they can make a robot brother.
Leo: Just tell them to get them a CI.

my helpful children

If you've got more than one child, balancing the needs of all the siblings is going to be one of the biggest challenges you'll face as a parent. Every one of your children, deaf and hearing, deserves the absolute best from you, all the time, and there's no possible way to make that happen. Navigating their different needs (without an army of clones) means finding the right compromises that won't shut your deaf kids out of family life or put unworkable burdens on your hearing kids.

Deaf and hearing siblings can open worlds for one another. Brothers and sisters are the first rivals, but also the first role models, informants, and collaborators. My children are different from one another in ways far beyond their ears, and when they're not squabbling over the latest *Captain Underpants* book, they learn from those differences. But that can only happen when communication is open for the whole family.[3]

---

[3] I'm going to recommend *Deaf and Hearing Siblings in Conversation* again. A super important book for families with a mix of deaf and hearing children.

Older Hearing, Younger Deaf

Birth order matters—if your older children are hearing, adjusting to a new deaf sibling can be tough. Especially for kids more than a year or two apart, adjusting to new communication patterns in your family will be a challenge, on top of the time and attention any baby pulls away from parents, let alone a deaf or deaf disabled baby. When Oscar arrived, it was ultimately Leo who had to make the biggest changes to his life. And unlike boneheaded relatives or clueless professionals, you need to have infinite patience and forgiveness with your children as they feel their way through the new reality.

When welcoming a new deaf baby, or recalibrating expectations when you discover one of your kids is deaf, remember that you set the tone. What you do, how you regard their deafness and give them access in the family will have a huge influence on what your hearing child will understand about the situation, how they will act, and can have an impact on their relationship long into the future.

Being matter-of-fact and upbeat helps; if you treat your baby's deafness as an interesting and (sometimes) fun difference, that will rub off on your hearing kids. When explaining things to younger children, you need to keep it simple and practical:

> "The new baby is deaf. That means he can only hear a little bit."
> "If you want your sister to understand, use the sign like I showed you."
> "If he can't see you, you need to stomp on the floor so he knows you're here."
> "Remember, we say hello like this <waving>."

We tried to be very direct and literal in our discussions with Leo, who was three-and-a-half when his brother showed up. It still took a long time—years—for him to really get the difference between his and his brother's experience of the world. Young children are developmentally stuck in their own perspective: they need a huge amount of practice and a couple of extra years of brain development before they can start truly seeing (or in this case, hearing) things from other people's point of view. Even so, they can learn to *behave* in certain ways, even if they don't understand the reasons deep down. It was only a week or two after we learned Oscar was deaf that Leo started telling people, "You need to use your hands to say hi," but he still sometimes forgets that his brother can't hear him if they're having a fight.

Children can be incredibly caring and protective of younger siblings, too, and you might hit the jackpot and have an older brother or sister who's excited by the chance to care for the new baby and wants to learn how to do it "right." Be cautious of letting them bear too much of the burden—a kid like that really doesn't know what they're getting into. This is a long road, and it can be hard on even the most enthusiastic little helper.

Big Feelings for Them

Whether they welcome the new baby with open arms or go into full rivalry mode, every hearing sibling will need plenty of space for themselves, lots of one-on-one attention from parents, and time away from the "deaf project" to feel secure and cared for. Schedule specific time for each of your kids if you can, and be sensitive to the way your attention gets divided. You might be spending most of your waking hours with the baby, but if you can devise a relatively bulletproof hour of activity for your hearing kids where they know they have your undivided attention, that can help older children feel safe and supported. And that can help them see their brother or sister as less of a competitor.

Another key is to make sure there's real communication happening *between* your kids, and don't be too quick to ascribe conflicts to their hearing differences. Inevitably, you'll have times when they plot against you in perfect harmony, and times when your older ones are just exasperated or need space and completely cut them off. It's especially at those times when you need to remember that modeling and playing are more effective than explicit instruction—behave the way you want your child to behave. If you make a mistake with your deaf kid, acknowledge and correct it. If your hearing children are fed up with signing, or any other aspect of communication, find the joke or the game to pull them back in (see the section on games below) or recognize that they need a break from the new paradigm. You want the fights to be about the last popsicle, not communication breakdowns and mutual frustration.

For my kids, the conflicts tend to come when the very extroverted and very deaf Oscar is excited about something and not wearing his devices, and either wants to involve his older brother or wants to be involved in his older brother's projects. It's hard for Leo, the more reserved one, to let Oscar know he needs his space. If Leo doesn't feel confident in his signing, this can result in him slamming doors and making other *physical* attempts to get some privacy.

Oscar needs to be aware that Leo isn't always available at his every whim, and Leo needs to know that if he wants Oscar to leave him alone in a kind and nonviolent way, he'll need to clearly communicate. This means taking a second to compose himself and get his hands up, not just signing STOP STOP STOP STOP STOP (although that can be a good first step).

Big Feelings for You

You will also have some supremely shitty feelings, both about your kids and about the situation in general. Having a deaf kid has been one of the most stressful experiences of my life, but seething with rage, worry, or sorrow doesn't actually help your deaf *or* hearing children; it makes parenting a lot harder. Finding professional counseling and even medication can be important if your feelings are keeping you back from connecting with and caring for your kids. But I'm also going to put in a good word for faking it, at least a little bit.

Putting on a brave face doesn't solve every problem, but it can protect your babies from the extremes of adult emotion that they can't understand and aren't built to handle. Although kids' needs seem urgent (and they sure know how to *insist*), if you're feeling overwhelmed, you can always take a break. Let the baby cry. Be late for school. Make your doctors wait. Take a minute, take an edible, say a prayer, and remember that this is not forever and nobody is doomed; if you've gotten this far into the book, you already know that you have options, and that your worries for your deaf child and for your family are probably exaggerated. You're all going to be OK, so putting on a brave face will help you *feel* brave and help the easier times come sooner. And allowing your children to watch you self-regulate, be responsible for your own health and behavior, is a much better lesson than allowing them to see you fly off the handle and lose control.

Of course, having a supportive partner, family, and friends, or a big babysitting budget is crucial for this project because holding it together for kids is strictly a part-time affair. You need to have a united front in the house, and you need a place to go away from the house where you can have fully grown-up feelings—another reason a therapist and / or respite care from your child's IFSP comes in handy. If your family doesn't have a lot of backup, consider teaming up with other families and swapping childcare chores.

Deaf Buddies for Hearing Sibs

This is also a great reason to get to know Deaf adults. If you're feeling anxious or down about having a deaf child, nothing will shake off the gloom as quickly as spending a couple of minutes chatting or texting with Deaf people about their lives and interests. And spending time with Deaf adults and kids will help your hearing children understand things better, too. When we found a Deaf nanny for deaf Oscar, we made sure hearing Leo spent some time with her, too, doing ordinary nanny things. Since then, she's graduated to auntie, and we have her over for Christmas or go on picnics when the weather is nice. We also make sure Leo comes with us to the deaf school and community events he'd enjoy. Any time he could possibly have fun with Deaf folks, we include him.

Separating siblings can also be powerful: the absolute best situations for Leo are where he gets one-on-one attention from cool young Deaf people, completely apart from his brother. He idolized the twenty-something Deaf swim instructor we found for him last summer, and his ASL is better for it. He also came back from a summer ASL course bursting with pride about his skills and filled with facts about the Deaf community he was eager to share. Being apart from Oscar puts the focus on him and his needs and abilities. Take a look at Deaf camps that accept hearing sibs, Deaf mentor programs, after-school stuff like Deaf sports teams or scouting troops.

Older Deaf, Younger Hearing

This one can be easier. Having a deaf older sibling means the new baby will grow up with expectations already in place. As tiny language sponges, they can pick up ASL and communication strategies naturally, as long as you make sure to expose them. That might mean setting separate times to sign and to talk with your hearing child just as you would with a bilingual deaf child—hearing playtime, signing bathtime, or whatever. Again, setting expectations and modeling behavior are really potent; the more you do the thing, the more likely your hearing child is to pick up that habit, too.

But deaf kids with younger hearing siblings can experience jealousy, too, especially if they feel like the hearing baby gets to do special "hearing stuff" with hearing parents; older deaf siblings will need the same kind of time-and-attention carve-outs as older hearing kids. Keeping on top of inclusion is critical, too—no forgetting to set the closed captioning for the cartoons, always signing when the deaf sib's around, and no dinner tabling, please.

Lots o' Deaf Babies

For hearing families that have several deaf kids, the advantages are potentially big for the siblings. Barring a miraculous vasectomy reversal, my deaf son will always be outnumbered by the hearing folks in the household, but he has friends who have two or three other deafies sleeping over every night—and hearing parents who have had time to learn the landscape and get familiar with all the wrinkles. Second kids never had it so good, and I know of families with three and four deaf children where the support and mutual understanding are just spectacular.

But there's an important caveat: parents can sometimes get snookered by older siblings when they apply the same model to their younger siblings. Genetic causes of deafness aren't always consistent in their effects. Hearing levels, anatomical quirks, and other aspects of deafness will vary kid-to-kid, not to mention the fact that our children are all individuals, with varying preferences and abilities that go way beyond their genes. Not getting complacent is important because there are no reruns in human reproduction.

I remember meeting a family one day out on the playground. I was signing with Oscar, and their very sweet 4-year-old came over to me, dragging his parents along. The kid was deaf and wore a cochlear implant. But he was over the moon to spot another adult who signed; his mother told me that she was the only one in the family who knew any ASL, and she mostly interpreted for him.

The boy's older brother was also deaf and had gotten a CI as an infant. Now, he was attending mainstream first grade and had age-appropriate English skills. This boy, though, who got his CI at the same age, was obviously struggling with language deprivation. His mother said he had about a 100-word vocabulary in ASL and a handful of words in English—way behind the expected total for a four-year-old. His father said they couldn't figure it out; his kids both had the same genetic condition and did the same therapies and interventions. They just kept waiting for the CI to "work."

I haven't seen them again, but I think of that kid often.

Kitchen Table ASL Games

If you're learning sign with your family, games at dinner time are a fun way to practice together and get hearing siblings moving their hands. It's also a surefire way to include your deaf kid in something fun at mealtimes if your small talk needs work.

Here are a few our family has found that are easy and work for many skill levels. These are all fast and simple, and the only rule I'd suggest enforcing is going voices-off for the duration of the game, even if your deaf child isn't participating. It can be tricky—younger kids will have a tough time code-switching, and older kids can get frustrated—but it's something to build toward. But the goal is, above all, to *play*.

I Spy: it's an easy game to start with because it uses so much of the vocabulary, classifiers, and spatial grammar that you learn in beginning ASL. In the unlikely event you've never played, one person has the job of "spy-er" starts the round by picking out something in the room and signing "I spy something green" (or whatever the color the object is). Then everyone takes turns guessing what the green thing is. Once someone correctly guesses the object, the role moves to the next person. That's it. You can keep score if you want, but with kids, there's usually no point—you go until everyone wins at least one round or they lose interest.

The great thing about I Spy is that it scales well for your children's cognitive development and your family's ASL skills. You can start using colors for clues and picking familiar objects—a red apple, a white chair, a green shirt, and so on.

But depending on where everyone's at with their age and their signing, you can move on to other types of clues: "something that's a circle," "something heavy," "something made of wood," and so on. Or you could use only ASL classifiers as clues, describing the shape of the object without any other nouns or adjectives.

It's also great with spelling and letters: "something that starts with the letter A," "something that starts with TH," and so on. We began learning ASL right around the time my hearing son was learning to read, and fingerspelling turbocharged his literacy skills.

20 Questions: All Q&A games are good for similar reasons, but unlike I Spy, a game like 20 Questions can involve more full sentences and conversational language. You can dial up the difficulty as you become more fluent and pick topics that match your kid's interests: favorite food, cartoon characters, prime numbers, whatever. One good variation is "I'm thinking of an animal," where you describe the place the animal lives, what it eats, how it moves, or whatever, and the kids try to guess. I do that one a lot through the car windows when I'm filling up at the gas station.

Waffle Doctor is barely a game at all, but it's fast and funny, and perfect for encouraging hearing siblings to expand their vocabulary. It started from a mistake I made: one day at breakfast, my attempt to sign DOCTOR APPOINTMENT went horribly wrong, and my kids thought it was the most hilarious thing on earth.

Start out by naming a food and a profession: WAFFLE DOCTOR, PANCAKE PLUMBER, and so on. Then your child does approximately the same thing: YOGURT DOG, COFFEE BOXER . . . whatever makes them laugh. You just go back and forth, around the table. Kids will rise to the challenge and want to learn new words to create the silliest combinations of them all; have your ASL dictionary on hand for lookups because POOP JUGGLER is classic. Obviously, you don't have to stick with the food + profession format; it's just a good place to start.

You can add an extra challenge to the game by trying to make visual rhymes using signs with the same handshape or body placement—MOOSE DAD, VOMIT MOM, and so on.

Handshape Challenge is just what it says. The first person picks one of the fifty-odd ASL handshapes and then challenges the rest of the table to come up with words that use the handshape. The role of quizmaster moves around the table. For this one, it's useful to have a stack of handshape flashcards to draw from or another reference so you can keep the game fresh.

Classifier Slapstick is a chance to express your inner Bugs Bunny (or Elmer Fudd). Kids take turns describing the funniest scene they can imagine in ASL: a person gets pushed off the edge of a cliff by a moose. An opera singer opens her mouth wide, and a bird flies in. Two kids are bouncing on the bed, and they accidentally jump to the moon. The possibilities are endless (but usually involve a person shoved from a high place).

You can also take turns adding to the story, so the first person sets up the joke ("I was about to eat a slice of pizza when . . .") and then the next person delivers the punchline (". . . the mushrooms punched me in the face!"). Like Waffle Doctor, this hardly qualifies as a game: the only point is to make something funny together.

Parents and Partners

If you're in a relationship, having a deaf kid is your ride-or-die moment. If you don't team up, raising a deaf baby can easily become the divorce maker. It's not just the work of childcare and appointments—you need to get clear on exactly how you'll make decisions for your child. Even an inch of daylight between you and your partner can end in a screaming match at the IEP meeting (and you can kiss your sex life goodbye). If you're separated from your partner, sharing custody means trying to build that united front for the kid—even if it's from behind a pane of bulletproof glass.

Every couple makes the pact differently, but every couple needs to start by talking; set aside a few minutes before assessments, meetings, and appointments, and agree on what your plan is. Right or wrong, pros like doctors and administrators can be hard to push back against. You'll have a much easier time if you both know what you want and what you're going to say beforehand. If it's a big meeting, talk the night before and make notes. Then, if something happens at the appointment where you need to change course, call a time-out and discuss with your sweetie in private—the *IEP Quick Start* chapter has more about meeting tactics.

Making decisions requires sustained energy and attention, and emotional durability when your bets don't pay off. You and your partner's capacity is going to wax and wane depending on your health, work situation, and the position of the earth's magnetic field, so there's no shame in sometimes delegating to one parent or another. But that delegation comes with responsibilities, too—you still need to sit down and talk over your plans, and you need to fully back each other once you've agreed, however you've agreed.

When we discovered Oscar was deaf, my wife was recovering from her pregnancy. She was exhausted, emotional, and in pain, and pouring through scientific papers full of worst-case scenarios and messy surgical pictures wasn't in the cards. So she sent me to do the first round of research while she nursed the baby and worked on healing. I told her what I found, without gory details, and what I felt was the best thing for Oscar, and we started from there.

Once she was back on her feet, our dynamic became 50/50. These days, we regularly have bedtime meetings about details in Oscar's IEP and related stuff where we talk over our options and our strategy equally. But sticking to the pact is still critical: if one of us needs to make a decision and the other one isn't around, we don't second-guess each other. At appointments, at school, and in front of the district, it's always *us*.

Dads and Other Dads

Sharing the load can be a challenge because in many opposite-sex couples, the woman becomes the caregiver by default, making all the decisions, booking all the appointments, and attending them with the baby. Not only can this arrangement get old real fast for mom, it's going to end up locking dad out of critical information, experiences, and relationships he'll need if he's going to have a say in raising his child. And before you go patting each other on the back, same-sex couples aren't immune to this dynamic, although y'all are usually more aware of it.

Even if one parent is the primary caregiver, you should both try to bring your kid to a few appointments solo. It helps the non-primary parent get a sense of what's going on and establish a one-on-one relationship with the professionals on your child's team. After all, if you only see the speech therapist at the IEP meeting, you're not really going to know what they're talking about, and it will be an uphill battle convincing them you know what *you're* talking about. Some dads describe feeling invisible when mom is in the room with a professional—all the attention can get directed toward the primary, which makes it even harder for the other parent to fully participate. This is less likely to happen if you've sat in on some solo visits with the SLP.

On the other hand, if you're the non-primary partner and you're feeling ignored by your kid's treatment team, going into a meeting or appointment alone is a great way to force everyone to pay attention to you. It also shows that you have your partner's trust and you're both in it to win it.

Attending appointments with your child is important in another way—nobody loves sitting through an endless session of booth testing at the audiologist, but doing it with your child lets them know you're in their corner and gives you a chance to see and experience a big part of their life. Even if you're the breadwinner and you can only make it once a year, it's worth sacrificing a sick day for it; your kid is only going to grow up once, and being there for the dull, painful, or scary bits is going to support your child and grow your relationship with them in ways you can't even guess at now.

Couples can also use unequal treatment to buffer and support one another. People comment on the most petty shit to my wife that they would never in a million years say to my face. So if you're "the mom," male or female, in a situation where you don't want to face down a lecture from some bigoted administrator, you can always send "the dad" in there alone for a five-minute, "sign this document and you're all set, sir."

It's Not About You, Bro

Splitting the "deaf chores" is especially important around learning sign language. Some parents—usually but not always fathers—can feel pressure to be the hero of the family and an effortless master of whatever challenge they face. Weirdly, this means that fathers are a lot *less* likely to put in the hours they need to learn ASL; it's really common to see families where moms are the only parent who signs.

The problem is that nobody's instantly good at a new language. These are complicated things that can only be learned gradually, with a huge amount of trial and error. You're not always going to be the best student in the room; you're going to need help at times, and you're going to make some embarrassing mistakes ("We can go home and fart together"). I've seen this fear—of failing, of needing help, or of looking ridiculous—keep plenty of dads, and some moms, away from ASL classes and Deaf social events.

I'm not immune. I would get intensely jealous during my wife's maternity leave. I was busy caring for our older son and working full days. She was at home with the newborn and her ASL book. Soon, she was chapters ahead of me, and it looked like I was never going to catch up. I'd come home every day and have to choke back my envy. It didn't help that she's got a doctorate in biology, so she's basically a learning machine with sexy legs.

Eventually I had to step back and understand that there was no point in being competitive. This was not a contest—or if it was, winning just meant that my family was happy. For them to be happy, I needed to be happy. If I was gonna be happy, I needed to know that this whole ASL thing was not about me.[4]

On top of this, unless you're married to a tradwife influencer, the non-caregiving partner is probably also the one bringing home the bacon. Actually finding time to take sign language classes may be hard or impossible if it's your job that pays the rent, but you can't let that be an excuse for not learning. There's a huge difference between *not learning* and *learning more slowly*. Having a demanding job means that you're going to have to find other ways to get ASL in the free time you've got—practicing at Deaf events on the weekends or squeezing in a ten-minute lesson on your phone at lunchtime. You don't need to be the hero, you just need to make progress.

Doin' It (Calendar Style)

Also, don't forget to have sex. Having a baby, especially a baby with special needs, can make one or both of you feel like you're strictly in survival mode. But as long as everyone is physically well and psychologically ok, it pays to make a plan and bang it out every once in a while.

---

[4]Of course, I wrote this book, so . . .

And I'm serious when I say "make a plan." I strongly recommend agreeing on a specific date, putting it in your calendar, and taking steps to ensure that you'll both be awake and available when the time comes. Because babies love chaos and hate your sex life, you may not actually get to smash, but make a good faith effort and do rain checks when it falls through. If fooling around at midnight seems too exhausting or impractical, find some afternoon care and book a hotel room.

Don't pack the fursuit or expect many handstands. Unless you guys first hooked up in the Olympic village, this is going to be low-energy maintenance sex. But maintenance sex is real and useful to remind you both why you had a baby in the first place. It's fully adult time when you step out of your role as parents and return to being lovers, caring for one another above anything else.

And if you're just too tired, try falling asleep in each other's arms.

Extended Family

Sadly, it's common for deaf children and adults to feel left out of things like holidays, reunions, and other gatherings. Even for kids who have access to spoken language, it's often impossible to understand what's happening in an ocean of voices and crosstalk. Whatever skills your child will acquire for speech, using their devices, and lip-reading are not going to make up for the fact that at a noisy barbecue, everyone might as well be playing kazoos.

At these events, dinner table syndrome cuts deaf children off from their roots, deprives them of the love and support of their extended family, the wealth that their home culture offers, and it's the last thing we want for our babies. Just like in your day-to-day life, there's no single solution to dinner table syndrome at family gatherings, just tactics.

Uncles, Aunts, Cousins, and Grandparents (Hearing)

Making sure your kid is included in family visits will mean different things; but above all, it will mean confronting your asshole brother-in-law. All the same anti-dinner table strategies that apply to your day-to-day life apply to bigger gatherings, but you've got to get your extended family on the same page with you.

Relatives can be uncomfortable accommodating deaf kids for a lot of reasons. There's ignorance about deafness, a lot of unspoken beliefs about the superiority of speech over sign language, tons of embarrassment, contrariness and control issues, and above all, a desire not to change the way they've always done things.

Your child will likely be the first deaf person they've ever really known, so whatever you ask of them *will* be an adjustment. Relatives who aren't visiting regularly aren't going to give your communication strategies the attention you give them, and nobody's going to get it right on the first try. There will be plenty of reasonable (and stupid) questions asked along the way, so be prepared to answer them with a little patience and grace. Every stupid question you answer now will be another stupid situation your kid won't have to face in a decade or two.

Remember that just like children, adults will get less frustrated and have fewer temper tantrums when you've given them a preview of what's going to happen, so preparing for a visit or holiday means sharing your expectations ahead of time. Send a note or have a conversation before the big day, and be simple and direct in what you expect:

> "Here's a list of signs you can use with the baby. I'm happy to do a Zoom with you if you need to go over them with me."
>
> "We're going to set up a TV in the back room this year. My kid can't hear the conversation if the game is on."
>
> "Hey, he won't understand you if you're not facing him. If he can't see you, you've got to tap him on the shoulder."

Age is no obstacle. Older relatives are sometimes excused because they're "from another time" or "set in their ways," but elders should be more sensitive to this than anyone—after all, they're probably losing *their* hearing, and turning on closed captions is going to help them just as much. Take a peek into an average adult-ed ASL class, and you'll see plenty of students over fifty learning sign for themselves, their spouses, or friends. If all else fails, you can always remind them that learning a second language delays the onset of dementia by up to five years.

Language Lessons for Late Learners

If your child uses ASL, it's completely reasonable to ask that your friends and extended family learn some sign language. And if your child relies primarily on ASL to communicate, having a functional vocabulary is essential if grandma ever wants to babysit. It's not too much to ask, and the barriers for learning these days are low as hell: at this moment, classes are available in person or online in every part of the country, at no or low cost.

Set your expectations on a spectrum: if you only ever see auntie Gina for Diwali, but she arrives with a dozen signs committed to memory, that's something to celebrate. But if uncle Greg is over for Sunday dinner every week, he'd better learn more than just HI and BEER in short order.

Give friends and relatives plenty of opportunities to learn and practice with you, and recognize their effort. As you know, language learning takes time, it can be emotionally tough, and they will likely never expend the effort you will—the stakes for them are fundamentally lower. But they'll have a better chance of sticking it out if you give them cookies along the way. Praise them for their effort, don't nitpick their signing, and give them opportunities to be with your child. The ultimate cookie, of course, is a relationship with their own flesh and blood, the cutest deaf kid in the entire universe.

Interpreters at the Funeral

Getting friends and family to play along is easier if you're hosting—your house, your rules—but it applies everywhere from Grandma's place to your cousin's destination wedding venue. Of course, being a guest means that you can't *force* accommodations; but getting in touch before the big event and making it clear what your child needs to be able to participate will give your host the opportunity to set up that access.

As your child gets older, an important strategy might be to hire an interpreter for big "hearing" holidays, family reunions, and such. Although it can seem strange to bring a professional into your private events, if your kid uses ASL, what you're really doing is bringing your *child* to these events in a complete way. You can offer to split the fees,[5] but keep in mind that for something like a wedding, a few hours of interpreting is going to cost your host less than the silverware rental.

In the end, accommodations, whether you're paying for a 'terp or just tweaking the seating chart, aren't "special"—they're basic to the event. If your relatives can't figure out a way to include your child, make plans not to attend. You don't need to be nasty or disappointed, just let them know that if they can't make it work, you'll catch them at the next thing. Standing up for your kid is critical because you're shaping your child's expectations for the future. Show them that access is their right, and that's what they will grow up believing. Setting boundaries is no fun, but it will quickly determine who actually gives a fuck about your child and who's only there for the macaroni salad.

Uncles, Aunties, Cousins, and Grandparents (Deaf)

Heredity plays a big role in deafness, so if you've got a deaf baby due to something like the GJB2 gene, yours might not be the only one in the family. If you have Deaf relatives that you don't know well, now might be a good time to get in touch. For all the reasons I've already stated, Deaf adults are often not in contact with their extended hearing families, and they may be delighted at a chance to renew relationships with you and your child and share their wisdom (and maybe a slice of pie at Thanksgiving).

It can be intimidating to reach out if you haven't been in contact, but it's well worth the effort. Text messaging, email, and interpreted video calls are more available than ever, making it easy to connect. Cousin Joy was the first person to give our family a Deaf perspective on growing up; she knew what our baby needed, and as we've continued on our journey, we're seeing how right she was and how lucky we were to get that insight from the beginning.

---

[5]There's a great discussion of adult siblings pooling the cost of an interpreter for family events in *Deaf and Hearing Siblings in Conversation*—a very important book on long-term Deaf-hearing family dynamics. If you want to know what your kids will think of each other after you're dead, this is the book to read.

Guest Signers and Chosen Family

If your child primarily uses ASL, another big way to make holidays more accessible is getting them together with other signers. If you have other Deaf or ASL-savvy relatives, make sure they're invited and seated together with your kid. If there aren't any Deaf cousins or signing uncles, consider inviting their deaf friends from school, so there's someone to talk to and celebrate with. I've even been to parties where there were separate signing and speaking rooms, if you're up to hosting a big crowd.

You can also consider consecutive or alternating celebrations. That could be a Deaf Thanksgiving followed by a hearing Christmas, or having your first night of Passover at the Deaf havurah, and the next with hearing relatives. If you do end up hosting a "mixed" event, remember that when inviting Deaf friends or relatives to your home, the onus is on you as the host to do your best to accommodate them and sign with them. You don't have to act as an interpreter the whole night, but make sure to include Deaf guests in the games, gift-opening, prayers, and so on, and spend equal time socializing with the Deaf and hearing sides. It can be easy to get caught up with the speaking crowd, but neglecting your Deaf guests is super rude. Also be aware that it's not every Deaf adult's dream to be the designated conversation partner for a two-year-old niece or their ASL newbie parent, so don't sweat it if your invitations aren't always accepted.

Weird Experiences for Hearing Parents Learning ASL

- trying to sign to hearing people over the phone
- trying to sign to hearing coworkers over Zoom
- having your first sex dream in ASL
- having your deaf kid figure out you're tapping the rhythm of the Muppet Show theme on his headboard to wake him up in the morning
- fingerspelling the nonsense poem that goes along with your kid's favorite "toothbrush video" and having him speak it back to you while he brushes his teeth
- going to the PTA meeting at the deaf school and having no idea who's Deaf[6]

---

[6] The Deaf parents know.

- switching to sign when your kid takes off their devices in the middle of music class
- going for a drink after ASL class and scaring the shit out of German tourists at the bar when you and your wife suddenly switch from signing to speaking

Testers and Doubters

Unfortunately, hearing relatives sometimes go completely haywire when presented with a deaf baby. This goes way beyond basic disagreements over sign versus speech or grumpiness about accommodations: it's a pathological reaction where they begin to act out against your kid in ways that are truly harmful and nuts. It seems to happen for a variety of reasons: your baby's arrival can undermine their sense of personal safety—"I won't ever go deaf!"—or challenge existing power dynamics in the family—"You had to go ahead and have that *special* kid!" or even insult their lineage—"Mutation?!? Our seed is PURE!"

This can create a sad phenomenon where family members either deny that your kid is deaf or continually test them to "prove" that they aren't. Either way, it's pathetic for them, painful for you, and can be very damaging for your child. Managing these types will take strong boundaries and some judicious elder abuse.

Testers seem to be trying to manage the panic they feel over being related to, or just being around, a deaf child. They'll call your child's name from behind, knock on pots and pans, and jump on any response they get as *proof* your kid can hear. Now, you probably did some amateur audiology early on, too, but hopefully you're not constantly re-running that particular experiment. Testers don't take your word for it, and they will keep pushing until they get the reaction they're looking for.

Doubters are generally making a straightforward power play. If your child is "really hearing," then they're right and you're wrong, they're smart and you're stupid, they can act however they want, and you need to ignore the harm they inflict. This can range from pure denial—"Oh no, she understands me," or "She's not deaf, just stubborn"—to more subtle undermining like, "She can *always* read my lips," or "The hearing aids work *perfectly*."

Both types will relentlessly exploit the ambiguity of baby communication and strategically dummy up when you try to explain the nuances of technology, hearing frequencies, language acquisition, etcetera. Evidence doesn't work: parents have pulled their kids' audiograms only to be told that the doctors must be wrong. Experts don't matter unless they agree with whatever the tester or doubter thinks. *Your* experience certainly doesn't hold any water, let alone your *kid's*.

When dealing with truly broken relatives like this, remember that it's not about deafness, it's about leverage. Whether they wrap their comments with "concern for the child" or just engage in straightforward aggression, this kind of behavior shows that they don't care about you, and they certainly don't care about your child. Overriding your experience and ignoring your kid's needs is the *whole point*.

In this situation, the only real control you have is your presence. Family members can go through a certain amount of denial, and they might never be Perfect Hearing Allies, but if they don't wise up reasonably fast—I say give them a year—then you'll need to limit visits. Never leave your child in the care of one of these people if you can help it.

Cutting Ties

Hopefully, as your baby grows up, practice will help your extended family get more comfortable socializing and communicating with them. Just know that there's a difference between slow on the uptake and willfully ignorant. About ten percent of everyone, and twenty percent of *your* family, are contrary dicks who will make it a point to thwart even modest attempts to include your child. Dealing with repeat offenders can be tough; there are only so many times you can remind adults of simple rules and basic decency, and even "good" family members can bend over backwards to justify or support the shitheads among you.

If your extended hearing family is especially stubborn or stupid and can't bring themselves to accommodate your kid after a year or two, stepping away from these jokers and finding your chosen family is important. Raising a healthy child means surrounding them with people who respect and cherish them for who they are and cutting off the people who demean and devalue them, even if they're your own parents.

"But Will," you might ask, "wasn't the last chapter about how connecting to their extended family is going to empower your child? How does cutting off family members relate to *that*?"

The thing about connection is that it's a live wire. It can bring you light, information, and warmth. Or it can shock your heart, fry your brain, and set your house on fire. If that connection hurts you every time you make it, you need to decide how much you're willing to suffer. More importantly, how willing you are to let your kid suffer before you cut the power?

The Fadeaway

This is the lowest-conflict route to take—just see the relative less. As they say, this ain't an airport and you don't have to announce your departure. It can be as simple as planning fewer events with them. Maybe you have a better side of the family you can prioritize for get-togethers, or maybe you can make it down to Disney World a little more often? Having a child is time-consuming anyway, so there's an element of plausible deniability baked into the tactic. It can exploit your relative's discomfort with your baby—shitty as it is, seeing less of you and your kid can be a relief to them. It's marvelously passive-aggressive, and depending on your family dynamics, the fadeaway might be enough to phase out bad actors entirely, or just serve to limit your child's exposure to them to tolerable levels.

It's nice if it works, but the fadeaway requires at least a little cooperation from the bad relative, and avoiding conflict just leaves it there as a booby trap ready to go off at an inconvenient time, like probate court. Relatives who are more aggressive in seeking you out, or who are more interested in abusing rather than avoiding you and your child, need other tactics.

The Honest Answer

If the problem relative is someone who's closer to you, whom you see more frequently, or who is especially toxic, you might have to be explicit as to why you're skipping their Arbor Day tree-planting party:

> "You made fun of her speech at the restaurant."
>
> "It's been a year and you haven't learned any ASL."
>
> "When we get together, you never face the baby when you talk."
>
> "Last time, you didn't bother to include our kid in anything."

Stating your case plainly and putting the burden where it belongs—on the asshole in question—is critical. You don't need to make a full accounting, just the appalling highlights. It's important to stick to the facts because this asshole has already proven they're not interested in how you feel, or they're interested in making you feel *bad*. Letting them know exactly how hurt you or your child are isn't going to help.

Email and text are good tools for this, because you can block / ignore / send replies to spam. If they're real bullies, you don't want to open yourself up to more abuse, and if they're real liars, you don't want to listen to more false promises. You've already invested twelve to twenty-four months, and you don't owe anyone—not a parent, sibling, or close friend—a conversation if they aren't arguing in good faith. Have a spigot you can close.

The honest answer has the virtue of being true, and you can repeat it to other relatives who want to know why you're not around. If those other relatives accept your reasoning, hooray! If they don't, well, now they know why you're not calling *them* anymore, either. The honest answer also models adult-level conflict-resolution skills for your kids. This is the response that comes from your best self, the parent who can defend your child, who gives respect even when the respect isn't returned, and who knows when to walk away.

It's also the tactic that requires the most self-control, because if you've come to this point, you're more than likely going to get an obnoxious reply. Your relative will tell you that you've hurt *their* feelings, or flip it around and give you some bullshit about how logical they're being and how hysterical you are, or any of a million other things. You will need to restrain yourself. Look and pass on, or just don't look at all. Given the *very small* amount of consideration you're asking for, they're not likely to ever change, and if they truly want to do better, your absence is the final warning. Let them enroll in some ASL classes and put the work in, then call you back later.

The Blowup

The last option is a fight. If you feel the need, you have my permission to throw a huge cathartic shit fit. It isn't your best self, but we're not always our best selves, and this is your kid we're talking about here.

Just be warned that while they feel good in the moment, fights are a calculated risk as a breakup strategy. A screaming match opens the door to false equivalence and accusations that you're being unreasonable, unrealistic, or especially if you're a woman, hysterical, and that has the potential to turn off other family members that you might otherwise keep on your side. On the other hand, if they're swayed by a fight with an abusive family member, were they ever worth keeping on your side to begin with?

Fights also have a nasty tendency to give the shittier party what they want. A certain type will want to see you upset and will be satisfied if you lose your cool. A dyed-in-the-wool narcissist will love a fight because it re-centers *them* in the argument instead of your kid. This kind of person will seek you out after the fight and try to provoke you again—set up the pins for another round of emotional bowling.

Fights can also lack finality; there are people out there who like to fight because then it obligates you to make up with them, or at least consider the issue settled. And in families that fight all the time, your attempt to truly end things might just get seen as a bump in the road. So if your family culture is like this, fights might be the first thing you do, but won't make sense if you really want to cut ties.

Ultimately, if you need to cut off a family member, no matter how you do it, I urge you to do it. Family are the ones who have your back. If they don't, they're not family. Ditch the relative, burn those bridges, and get to work building new ones.

Family Heritage (Matzah Balls, etc.)

Back in the 90's, my father brought my then-80-something grandmother to an ASL class. This was decades before his deaf grandson was born—he was taking the class to connect with his mom's experience.

Both of my grandmother's parents had been Deaf, and she had grown up in New York City in the 1910s and 20s, interpreting for them in their day-to-day interactions. This doesn't happen anymore, except in movies, but before the Americans with Disabilities act, being the interpreter-child was a fact of life for some CODAs.

Although she'd grown up signing, she had gone on to marry a hearing man and hadn't signed much in the decades since her parents passed away. My father knew her history and was curious how much sign language she remembered.

A lot, as it turned out; much of what she'd always thought were her family's "home signs" were really a time capsule of early 1900's ASL. The Deaf teacher was amazed and delighted. In true Deaf culture fashion, he began quizzing her about her parents:

How did they meet? Where did they go to school? How did they arrive in New York? And then,
"Their families came from Russia? Why did they come to America? Were they looking for better jobs?"
She looked at him like he had three heads:
"Why did they come from Russia? They were killing the Jews!"

We are all more than one thing. Your child will never just be deaf; they will be Jewish and deaf, Black and deaf, LGBTQ+ and deaf, and so on. Having access to their culture, communities, and traditions is going to support and enrich their lives. Culture doesn't just mean knowing what food to cook or what level of sarcasm to use. Culture is a survival kit—this is why there's a "big-D" Deaf culture to begin with. But Deaf culture isn't the *only* culture that has tools for your child. Knowing who you are gives you strength and strategies to face the world and fight for what you need.

Your kid will need to fight; send them out fully armed.

Already Here

Deaf children are born into every family on earth, so if you look, it's almost certain that you'll find your people already present inside the larger Deaf community. In the United States, there are organizations and resources for Deaf people of many backgrounds. Through them, your child can find peers and mentors, and grow up knowing the history, achievements, and contributions of folks who are like them in more ways than just being Deaf.

We are talking about communities within communities, so finding your Deaf roots may involve more networking and travel than just connecting to the local Deaf crowd. The Internet, as always, has made things easier, and I strongly encourage you fall down the Google hole to find out more about Deaf people who share your family's heritage. I've included a few prominent figures from each community to give you a head start, with a bias toward people who are alive and interesting, but not necessarily child-appropriate or safe for work!

Still, there's no replacement for meeting people IRL; Deaf cultural organizations like Black Deaf Advocates or Asian Signers will often have holiday gatherings, presentations, and support for families and children. Many of these groups use social media to organize, so if you don't find much on their website, head over to Facebook, Instagram, or TikTok to see the latest.

On the topic of "deaf and . . ." it's important to acknowledge that plenty of folks have *multiple* identities, including the people I name below: Lauren Ridloff has both Black and Mexican heritage, Antoine Hunter identifies as both as Black and Native American, and Chella Man is Chinese and Jewish, as well as being a certified hunk. There is also a growing number of superheroes in the Deaf BIPOC community as well—I've marked them with an <s>, so please respect their secret identity.

Deaf Asian American and Pacific Islander Communities

The Deaf AAPI community has been organizing itself in the United States since the 1970s, with the founding of the National Asian Deaf Congress. These days, there are local, national, and international groups that celebrate the many cultures and traditions of Deaf Asian Americans, including Asian Signers and local groups like the Metropolitan Asian Deaf Association (NY) or the Bay Area Asian Deaf Association.

There are well-developed Deaf communities in some Asian countries as well, and parents looking to connect their children with their heritage can look to organizations overseas as well as in the United States.

Deaf Asian folks to look up:

Educator and writer Madan Vasishta (Indian American): Author of the autobiographical *Deaf in Delhi* and *Deaf in DC*, he is a professor at Gallaudet University in the United States and an activist for Deaf rights and Indian Sign Language in India.

Artist Christine Sun Kim (Korean American): A maker of epically snarky drawings, installations, and sound pieces focused on her life as a Deaf woman. She's written and presented on Deafness and other topics, and signed the national anthem at Super Bowl LIV.

<s> **Actor, artist and model Chella Man (Chinese American):** Also an author, director, VR programmer, they portrayed superhero Jericho on *Titans*.

Cartoonist CJ "Caldatelier" Reynaldo (Filipino): Prolific illustrator and cartoonist who publishes adorkable work in English about Deaf life in the Philippines, along with folklore, cute monsters, and how-to guides in American and Filipino Sign Language.

The Black Deaf Community

Like the hearing Black community, the Black Deaf community has a powerful culture rooted in the Black experience of segregation, tradition, and solidarity. The National Black Deaf Advocates has branches across the country and are a good place to begin for Black families looking for more information, but you should also look out for regional organizations like Bay Area Black Deaf Advocates.

Black American Sign Language

Although not all Black Deaf people use it, Black American Sign Language (BASL) is a distinct sign language that has been passed on through Black Deaf families and between peers for generations. Because BASL has retained some features and signs that have been lost to modern ASL, it's uniquely connected to the roots of American Deaf culture and language as a whole. If you're a Black family, a Black Deaf mentor can show you the ropes.

Some Black Deaf people to know:

Educator Carolyn McCaskill: Black Deaf history scholar, founding director of Gallaudet University's Center for Black Deaf Studies, and co-author of *The Hidden Treasure of Black ASL*.

<s> **Actress Lauren Ridloff:** A former teacher and Miss Deaf America, she's starred on Broadway, TV, and in the Marvel movie *Eternals* as the superfast superhero Makkari.

Influencer Nakia "itscharmay" Smith: BASL advocate and all-around TikTok superstar, as well as the BASL interpreter for the recent blockbuster *Sinners*.

Lawyer Haben Girma: The first DeafBlind attorney to graduate from Harvard Law—activist, Obama-adjacent person, and author of the bestselling memoir *Haben*.

Actor CJ Jones: The granddad of Black Deaf actors. You probably saw him in *Baby Driver*, or remember his legendary appearance on *A Different World* back in the day.

Comedian Sheena "MsDeafQueen" Lyles: Famous for roasting hearing clout-chasers on TikTok and Instagram who try and teach shitty ASL. She is merciless.

<s> **Musician and actor Warren "WAWA" Snipe:** Rap artist and creator of Dip Hop, and quietly magnetic screen personality. Appeared in *The Walking Dead* and *Black Lightning*. Signed the national anthem at Super Bowl LV.

Educator Laurene Simms: Chief Bilingual Officer at Gallaudet University and a highly respected scholar and researcher. Laurene is a huge advocate for language acquisition and development for deaf children.

The Deaf Latine Community

Latine people are the single largest minority group within the US Deaf community; in my son's class here in Northern California, about half the parents use Spanish at home. There are national organizations like Council de

Manos and the National Hispanic Latino Association of the Deaf, as well as statewide organizations like California's Manos del Corazón are all there for families to discover. LA-based Deaf Latinos Y Familias Organization is a must for families whose first language is Spanish.

ASL Lessons in Spanish

Families sometimes assume you need to know English before you can learn ASL, or can only find lessons or materials in English. Fortunately, there are increasing opportunities to skip the middleman and learn ASL with Spanish-fluent teachers and handouts. Besides the organizations listed above, some deaf schools, as well as the American Society for Deaf Children and ASL at Home, offer classes and curriculum books in Spanish. Perfect for getting *abuelo* up to speed.

LSM and Beyond

Latin America has an array of national and indigenous sign languages. Families who have contact with the Mexican Deaf community might encounter *Lengua de Señas Mexicana* (LSM) in particular. Parents looking to connect their children with their heritage can look to organizations in their home countries as well as in the United States.

Some prominent Deaf Latine personalities:

Journalist Melissa Elmira Yingst: Queen of the Deaf talk show, she keeps the community informed and entertained with her program *Melmira*.

Yashaira Romilus: DeafBlind educator and community leader with Puerto Rican roots, "Yash" is also a pioneer in ProTactile theater.

Influencer Estefani "thatdeaffamily" Arevalo: An advocate for ASL, a Deaf interpreter, and mother of two startlingly cute Deaf children whose lives she documents on social media.

Roberto Cabrera: A Dominican-born DeafBlind educator, councilor and Protactile trainer, and advocate for the DeafBlind community.

Comedians Jimmy Linares and Alvaro Garcia: Co-superstars of *Deafies in Drag*, the breakout Deaf comedy show of the 2020s. They slay.

Ivy Velez: A Puerto Rican-born community leader and educator with strong roots in the Latina Deaf community.

Native American and First Nations Deaf Communities

Deaf people have always been part of Native communities in North America, and different groups have their own traditions around deafness. You can find information and Deaf elders online at the Gathering of Deafatives, Turtle Island Hand Talk, or through your tribal government.

Indigenous Sign Languages

Today, most Deaf Native Americans, Hawaiian and Alaskan Natives and First Nations people use ASL, but there is ongoing interest in preserving indigenous Deaf traditions and sign languages. The best known is Plains Sign Language (PSL), which was once used as a common language by tens of thousands of deaf *and* hearing people across a huge swath of North America. There are efforts to revitalize PSL and other languages like Oneida Sign, Hawai'i Sign Language, and Inuit Sign Language in native communities and colleges.

Some Indigenous Deaf people to know:

Activist and educator Marsha Ireland (Oneida): The elder behind the reconstruction of Oneida Sign Language, she advocates for reclaiming indigenous Deaf identities.

Artist and activist Sarah Young Bear-Brown (Meskwaki): Founder of the Gathering of Deafatives, she is a community organizer and political person as well as a fifth generation beadworker.

<s> **Actress Alaqua Cox (Menominee and Mohican):** Actress who kicks ass with her prosthetic leg as the Deaf Disabled villain-turned-superhero Echo in *Hawkeye* and *Echo*.

Choreographer Antione Hunter (Cherokee and Blackfoot): World-famous dancer and head of Urban Jazz Dance Company, one of the leading Deaf dance troupes on the planet.

The List Goes On . . .

This is just a start for families looking for some reference points and role models; the world is filled with accomplished and talented deaf folks from every background doing just about everything. You can find links to more deaf folks at willfertman.com

Home Culture / Deaf Culture

In this book, I'm pretty much assuming that you speak English at home and will need to add ASL to the mix in one degree or another. But what if you speak Spanish at home, or Cantonese, or Navajo?

It's at this point that some idiot SLP or ToD will jump in and say, "Ah ha! THIS is why your kids need to hear and speak! To the Oralismobile!"

More reasonable parents may ask, "I want my child to know their heritage language so that they can know their roots, culture, and their extended family. How are they going to do that in sign language?"

That imaginary SLP is a numbskull, but the parents have a good point. Raising your kid with connections to their roots is a part of bringing up a healthy child, and finding ways to make your home or heritage language accessible can be important.

Because strong *language* skills are going to be the basis for all other learning for the rest of your kid's life, learning ASL doesn't exclude learning your home languages—quite the opposite. Giving your child a strong basis in sign language will ensure that you'll be able to pass on what's meaningful to you about your home culture, whether your child has access to speech or not. In fact, it's not unusual to run into multilingual Deaf adults who have a handful of languages that they can fluently sign, read and write, or speak. After all, if they were fortunate enough to get a solid bilingual ASL-English education as children, they started out *already bilingual* and benefited from all the cognitive advantages that bilingualism has, including more easily learning additional languages on top of their starting two.

This doesn't mean teaching your child your home language isn't challenging. Finding language models and making the arrangements for additional language learning can be daunting. Grandparents or other relatives sometimes carry unhelpful prejudices about deafness and might not make the best tutors. And some spoken languages, especially tonal languages like Cantonese or Yoruba, might be harder to perceive using hearing devices when compared with English.

And if your child doesn't have easy access to spoken language, you may have to shift gears. As one Deaf high schooler put it to me, "I took Latin because nobody cares about pronunciation." On the other hand, there are also Deaf communities and sign languages in your home countries, so learning Japanese Sign Language or *Lengua de Señas Mexicana* is another option to connect to your home culture, and the internet has created more opportunities for that than ever.

Religion

Because of their work in education and social support, faith communities have run parallel to Deaf communities since forever: it's no coincidence that Abbé l'Épée founded his school in Paris so his students could make confession, or that Thomas Gallaudet was an Episcopal minister. Raising your deaf child in your family's religion is absolutely possible—snoop around and you'll find accessible services and education for many faiths and sects, both in-person and remote. But you will need to do your research on finding appropriate churches, temples, and mosques that match your beliefs and offer more than superficial inclusion, and beware of predatory evangelists and others who look at deaf kids and their families as easy pickings.

Church Terps and Accessible Communities

Unlike other public organizations, places of worship are generally exempt from ADA rules around access for deaf people. Despite this, some institutions make it a point to have ASL interpretation available for services, but unfortunately, the quality can vary widely. While some church interpreters are professionals, skillful CODAs, or other fluent signers, others are well-meaning volunteers who can't handle more than the basics, if that. Church terps can feel very proud of their contributions and be very earnest in their desire to make services accessible, but that doesn't mean much if they're signing gibberish. If you bring your child to services, please don't be shy about insisting on quality interpretation.

And services are the tip of the iceberg. Even places that provide professional terps might only do so on Sunday morning (or Friday, or Saturday . . .). If you want your child to participate fully in the community, you will need to work to make sure religious education, youth groups, potlucks, and other events are accessible to them,[7] and delivered in ways that aren't ableist or audist—no begging for inclusion, no seating at the back of the congregation, no being singled out for "bravery" or "healing."

Any good priest, pastor, rabbi, or imam should be coming to you and to your kid, for guidance on how to include them in the life of the community. Unfortunately, ministers don't always practice what they preach, and they don't exactly hand out certificates in deaf studies along with theology degrees. It can be tough to leave a place you love, but if your home church can't or won't accommodate your child, you will need to make some decisions, and your best bet for full inclusion might be a Deaf-led congregation.[8]

A Word on Miracles and Faith Healing

Deaf babies are an awful temptation for certain faithful people. Sooner or later, *someone* will pray for your child to be "healed." In the rare moments I've encountered this, I just politely decline.

> Prayers seem harmless on the surface, but offering to pray for your deaf child in front of them implies that there's something wrong with them.
>
> It's a little thing, but it's a paper cut to a tiny and fragile self-esteem. If this happens many times during your growing years, you start to think—unconsciously or not—that something IS wrong with you. I wish my parents had pushed back forcefully each and every time.
>
> Molly, Deaf adult

As for laying on hands, please think twice. Deaf adults can have hellacious stories of faith healing attempts by strangers, family, and ministers, who regard "curing" deafness as the grand prix of miracles. This is often traumatic and confusing for kids, making a spectacle of them and risking alienation from you and your faith forever. If you value your child, their relationship with God,

---

[7] Religious texts, in particular, can be tricky for kids who have English as a second language. Locating quality signed scripture is important.

[8] Or possibly splitting time between your home congregation and and Deaf-led one.

and their relationship with you, don't do it and don't allow others to do it, no matter who they are.

See the chapter *Snappy Answers to Stupid Questions* for more on this one.

Missionaries: Don't Call Us, We'll Call You

Take it from this Jew, nothing's worse than being a notch on someone else's spiritual bedpost. Certain Christian sects are infamous in the Deaf community for aggressively pursuing converts, keeping records of folks in the community and sending missionaries repeatedly to their door. This is motivated by the mistaken belief that deaf kids somehow aren't taught about religion at home and are therefore ripe for recruitment. Of course, that will not apply to *your* family, because you've raised your child without dinner table syndrome, knowing all about their family's heritage and beliefs. If the same denomination keeps turning up like a bad penny, tell them to go get fucked and to take your name off the list.

This can go beyond doorknockers; you may run into people in various roles like interpreters or care workers who make it their business to proselytize on the job. This is almost always inappropriate and unethical; you and your child have the right to get services without scripture. You should report unwelcome on-the-job witnessing to managers and authorities because this behavior drives people away from services and makes it harder for deaf kids, adults, and their families to get the support they need. See *Dealing With Bad Professionals* for full details.

Christian Denominations

The Episcopal Church has deep connections to the American Deaf community and has been offering services in ASL since Thomas Gallaudet the Younger began ministering at St. Ann's in New York City in 1852. Gallaudet shares a feast day with the first Deaf clergyman in the United States, Rev. Henry Winter Style, celebrated on August 27. The Episcopal Conference of the Deaf has information on Deaf clergy and accessible services and ministry in the United States.

The Catholic Church maintains a network of offices and chaplaincies for Deaf people, with interpreted services available as well as a respected bilingual school, St. Rita's School for the Deaf, in Cincinnati, and a well-regarded summer camp with programs open to deaf kids of all faiths, Camp Mark7, in upstate New York. St. Francis de Sales is the patron of the Deaf, and his feast day is January 24. Check with the National Catholic Office for the Deaf for more information.

The Orthodox Christian Deaf Association was founded in 2020 as the first pan-Orthodox organization to connect Deaf Orthodox Christians "in order to foster fellowship, create useful resources, both educational and liturgical, plan special events, and to introduce the greater Deaf community to the Orthodox faith." St. Mark the Deaf is an Orthodox patron of Deaf people, and his feast day is January 2.

The Church of Latter-day Saints maintains lists of Deaf wards and branches, as well as educational materials in ASL, and a recently established ASL Board of Education to coordinate religious instruction for young people. You may have to dig around—the services were not well organized at the time of this writing.

For other Christian denominations, there are a variety of Deaf and accessible churches throughout the country from mainline to evangelical, delivering services and pastoral care. Some simply offer interpreted services, while others have Deaf ministers or offer full Sunday school instruction, summer camps, and other opportunities in ASL. Research is important: like all other Deaf services, word-of-mouth (sign-of-hand?) is going to be the best guide.

Judaism

Because of genetic factors (thanks Bubbie and Zayde!) deafness is somewhat more prevalent in the Jewish community than average, and Deaf Jewish organizations have come and gone over the years to serve that community. Because of our small numbers, finding an accessible or Deaf synagogue or rabbi in the neighborhood, or via remote, is harder than finding a church, but they're out there; look in communities with deaf schools and in larger cities. There's even an interdenominational Deaf rabbinical school in the United States, Hebrew Seminary. Organizations like the Jewish Deaf Congress, and the Jewish Deaf Resource Center have information on finding services, celebrating holidays, and getting accessible Hebrew schooling and Bar and Bat Mitzvah prep across the Orthodox-Conservative-Reform-Revival spectrum.

Islam

Like Jews, families in the Muslim ummah may have to search harder for accessible services and religious education for their deaf children, but it helps to be in a community with a large Muslim population. Nationally, The Deaf Muslim Association, Islamic Services for Deaf and Hard of Hearing, and Global Deaf Muslims are organizations with information and education for deaf Muslim kids and their families.

Other Beliefs

Families who follow other faiths will want to check online, with their local spiritual leaders, and with larger Deaf groups for information and fellowship—as always, Deaf community members are your best resource. Many less centralized groups like pagans or atheists organize via social media and can be found on Facebook and friends, so start digging.

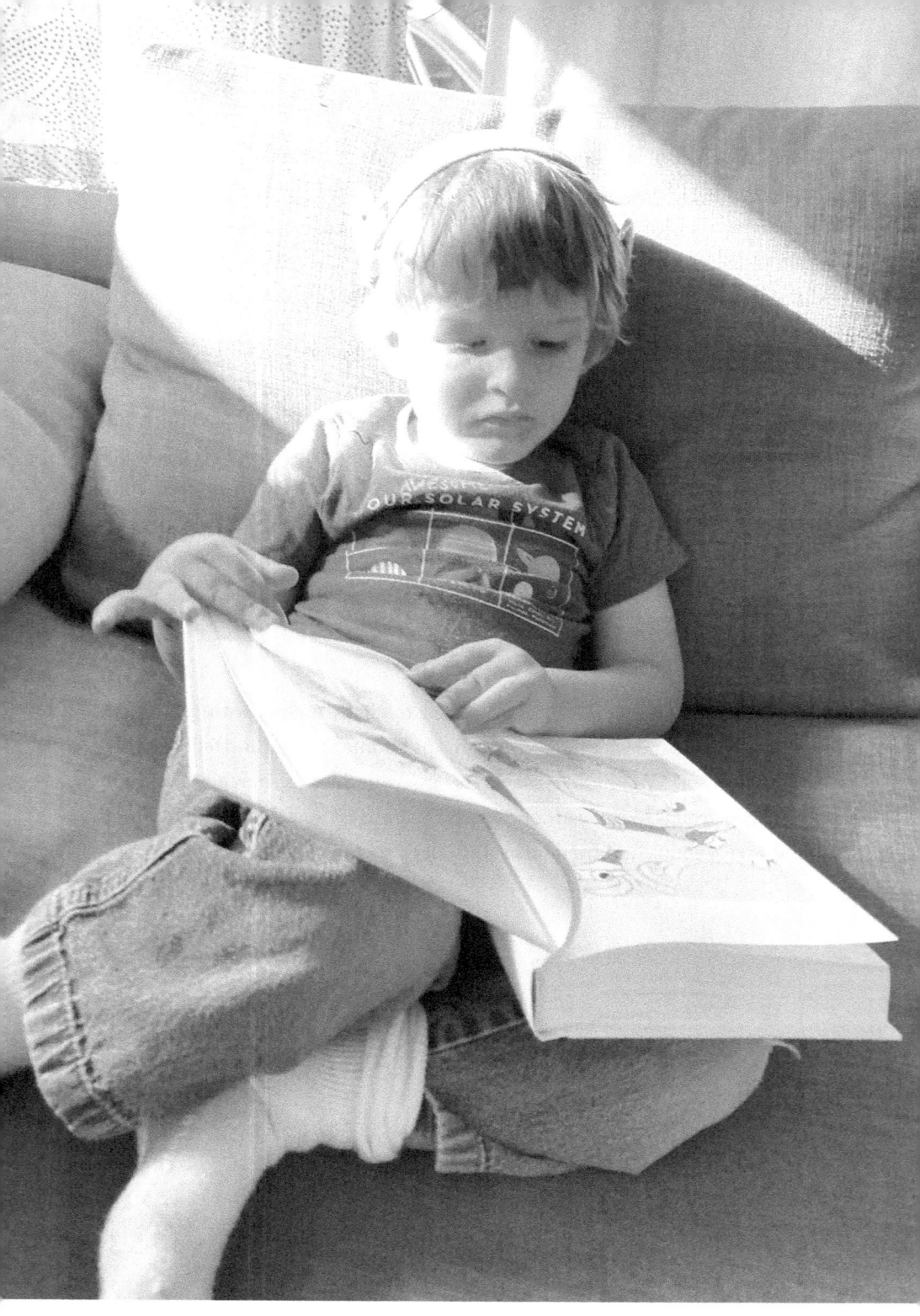

Will Fertman, 2025

4

Doctors, Teachers, and Assholes

These are the fun chapters about getting your deaf child therapeutic and educational services.

Sike.

As the hearing parent of a deaf kid in the United States, you will need to deal with our less-than-lovely medical and educational systems. Figuring out what medical interventions, if any, your child needs, and getting them done right, is one project. Figuring out what educational and therapeutic supports your child needs, and getting *them* done right, is a whole other project.

The good news is that there are entire government agencies dedicated to helping with this. The bad news is that the system has been distorted by a century-plus of bigotry and bad practices, and, at the time of this writing, is under vicious assault by the president and his administration. On top of that, no two hospitals or school districts are alike when it comes to deaf kids. You can have very different experiences based on what community you live in, what kind of insurance you can afford, and of course what color your skin is.

Individual educators, doctors, interpreters, and other professionals also play a huge role in accessing proper care and education for deaf kids—good ones are rare, and bad ones can make it seem impossible to get your child what they need. You can waste a lot of time stuck in a bad school district or with a bad professional and not even know what your options are.

This section of the book is my attempt at giving you the big picture—the details will change state by state and town by town. Deaf ed involves some truly hellacious bureaucracy, and there will be tons of acronyms, so B.U.C.K.L.E. U.P.[1]

Deaf Ed Is Not a Guy

Navigating a deaf kid's schooling is tricky because you've got to hit the ground running. The birth-to-three window for language acquisition means you need to move quickly to support your baby's development and start making decisions *fast*. The deaf education industrial complex doesn't give you a lot of help. There are still legions of hearing professionals out there wedded to disproven ideas about childhood language acquisition. Even if your doctor or audiologist is hip to pediatric deafness, there is a baked-in reluctance to make recommendations based on research in the name of professional neutrality. Deaf professionals almost always have a better grasp of the issues, but you'd be lucky as hell to run into one by accident.

To understand the landscape and start picking your best course of action, you need some critical pieces of background:

- the fucked up history of deaf education in the United States
- the educational methods, good and bad, that are still around in the wake of this history
- the natural languages and artificial sign systems these methods use, and what research says is best for your kid
- The different kinds of schools and programs that might be available, and the balancing act you'll need to perform to get your baby everything they need
- You and your child's legal rights to getting this education through the IFSP, IEP, and 504 process

So without further ado . . .

---

[1]Because yoU Can't Kill Language Enemies Under Penalty of law.

A Long and Boring History of Deaf Education in the United States

Quick, get the time machine… We need to kill the inventor of the telephone!

Deaf education in the United States has some high highs and low lows. Like education for a lot of minority groups, it's been shaped by bigotry and neglect, but also individual heroes and communal triumphs against long odds—and it ain't over yet. Ultimately, the Deaf community has shown that when they control their own institutions, deaf children can excel, and when it's good, America has the best deaf education in the world.

The very short story is this: starting in the early nineteenth century, America developed a robust network of boarding or *residential* schools that taught deaf children using ASL as the classroom language. This worked well overall, and the schools graduated several generations of educated and successful Deaf adults. Then, around 1900, the system got shredded by a coordinated campaign to legally forbid sign language and mandate speech and lip-reading in the schools, which undercut almost all the progress they'd made. At the same time, the spread of eugenics, a massively fucked-up social-political ideology, made it easier to write off deaf people as damaged goods. The aftermath was decades of struggle and pain for deaf kids, but between 1960 and today, Deaf political activism, cognitive science, educational research, and the legal system have slowly caught up with the realities of what makes a good deaf education.

Today, there are high-quality schools and programs out there, and strong rights to help you get the best education for your child. Sadly, the years of neglect and oppression have still left their mark. If you look out on the landscape of deaf education, you'll find programs that reflect almost every misstep and dead-end approach, many of them using outdated and disproven teaching techniques and still carrying biases rooted in Victorian-era pseudoscience. And as of 2025, the president has undertaken a sustained effort to destroy the federal supports for all these systems. So while your kid has a better chance at a quality education now than at almost any time in the past, bad options are still more common than good ones, and bad options may be the *only* options in your area.

This is a topic that's already consumed whole books, so I'm sticking to the key points. It might seem weird to be talking about higher education if you're looking at preschools now, but the changes trickle down, so knowing what happened at Gallaudet University in 1988 is going to help you understand what's going on at Sunshine Cottage today. Names and terminology have changed a lot over two-and-a-half centuries, so to keep things simple, I'm referring to existing schools and organizations by their current titles, using the modern names for all the sign languages, and the capital-D spelling of Deaf where appropriate.

1760–1817: *Vivre la France!*

Deaf education in America starts in France in 1760, when Abbé Charles-Michel de l'Épée, a hearing Catholic clergyman, founded what is now known as the National Institute for Deaf Children in Paris. This was the first free school for the deaf in all of Europe, and l'Épée set it up to give poor deaf kids a religious education. The idea was rooted in the Enlightenment philosophy prevalent at that time: all people were essentially rational, and if given the proper tools, they could use their reason to improve themselves. So if deaf children had access to language and information, they could confess their sins, take communion, learn a trade, testify in court, and participate in public life.

Abbé l'Épée started with what's now known as *Old French Sign* to teach, a language he learned from the Deaf community in Paris. He tried to add a lot of awkward features to make it more like spoken French, but the students at the school continued to use the original language outside of class. Eventually, as those kids grew up and became teachers at the school, they incorporated and adapted some of l'Épée's changes, notably the alphabet, creating a new language, *Langue des Signes Française* (LSF). With an accessible natural language, along with l'Épée's willingness to share his techniques, Paris became the center of sign language-based deaf education for the Western world.

Half a century later in 1814, across the Atlantic in Hartford, Connecticut, a hearing pastor named Thomas Gallaudet met a nine-year-old deaf girl named Alice Goswell. She was the neighbor's daughter and had no language or education up until that point. Gallaudet became interested in teaching her, and since there were no deaf schools in the United States, her family and some other locals funded a research trip to Europe to bring back modern deaf educational practices. When Gallaudet visited the Institute in Paris, he was impressed with the high level of achievement of the students, and he persuaded a Deaf teacher, Laurent Clerc, to come back to Hartford with him. Clerc brought LSF along and, with Gallaudet, founded the American School for the Deaf as a sign-language-based residential school in 1817.

1817–1880: Deaf Renaissance

What followed was an explosion in Deaf education in America. Hearing and Deaf families saw new opportunities for their children and sent them to live at the new school in Connecticut. The Deaf students brought their own local sign languages with them, and Clerc's LSF absorbed elements from these, creating a new American Sign Language.[2] Adults who had been educated in Hartford would go on to teach there or work at one of the newer residential schools that were founded across the country, forming a network of more than twenty sign-based schools in the United States and Canada by the mid-1800s.

The Deaf community began to organize itself with these schools at their core. While there were many obstacles for deaf children, the residential schools both provided a deep well of experienced teachers and a community that understood how to support them. Literacy for the average Deaf adult, which was very unusual before, began to climb rapidly. A child sent to live at the American School or another residential institution was likely to stay there through the twelfth grade, and in an age when many hearing kids left at grade six or eight to work, this meant that Deaf people were often the best-educated members of their family. By the time of the Civil War, an estimated forty percent of all teachers in the residential schools were Deaf themselves.

---

[2]Besides LSF, the greatest contributor to modern ASL is thought to be the now-extinct Martha's Vineyard Sign Language, as well as sign languages from communities in New Hampshire and Maine. It's *also* thought that Native American sign languages influenced ASL—and there's still more to learn. Check out *Everyone Here Spoke Sign Language* by Nora Ellen Groce for more on Martha's Vineyard Sign Language and the remarkable Deaf community there.

With access to language, education, and a widespread support network, Deaf adults had new opportunities. Deaf journalists like Laura Redden Searing interviewed politicians and generals for national newspapers, Deaf clergymen like Henry Winter Syle founded congregations, and Deaf artists like Douglas Tilden were celebrated (and scandalous!) public figures. And decades before Helen Keller became a celebrity, crowds were coming to the American School for the Deaf to witness DeafBlind women like Julia Brace defy expectations just by going about their daily business.

Finally, in 1864, Gallaudet's youngest son, Edward, successfully petitioned Abraham Lincoln to allow Washington DC's local residential school to award advanced degrees. This was the start of Gallaudet University, the first institution of higher learning for Deaf students in the world.

1880–1900: Oralism ♥ Eugenics

While sign language education was now the norm for most residential deaf schools in the United States, there were always families that wanted their children to speak and read lips. In 1867, Gardiner Greene Hubbard, a lawyer whose daughter had lost her hearing at age five, founded the Clarke School for the Deaf in Northampton, Massachusetts. Drawing on the support of the wealthy New England elite, it would go on to be the most influential oral program in America.

While oralism's dismal overall results were seen and criticized by educators and Deaf adults at the time, it would be more than a century before the process of language acquisition and the causes of language deprivation in deaf children were well understood. This was a problem because control of state-funded institutions lay largely in the hands of hearing politicians and bureaucrats who had no firsthand knowledge of the issues at all, creating a situation ready to be exploited by oral school supporters.

In 1880, the oralist Pereire Society organized the Second International Congress on Education of the Deaf in Milan, Italy. The Milan Conference was a carefully staged event, intended to create the impression of consensus among professionals that the oral method was superior. The delegates were drawn from the United States and across Europe, and selected for their beliefs—at a time when nearly half the teachers in deaf schools in the United States were Deaf themselves, there was only a single Deaf delegate, and only a handful of sign language advocates among the 164 attendees. This made the outcome easy to guess: a set of resolutions supporting deaf education, but opposing the use of sign language in schools. These resolutions became ammunition for oralist educators to "prove" oralism's superiority to authorities in the United States, and American lawmakers and administrators to mandate oral education in deaf schools.

But the Milan Conference wasn't the only factor that turned back the progress of deaf education. Social changes were happening rapidly in America throughout the nineteenth century and accelerated with the end of the Civil War in 1865. The emancipation of slaves, the arrival of new immigrants from Europe and Asia, and the rise of women's suffrage created fears in the American ruling class about maintaining their power and position. The response to this upheaval was a new, brutal social movement masquerading as rationalism called *eugenics*.

Eugenics was based on the growing awareness of the way traits like eye color are passed from parents to children, which was just beginning to be studied in a systematic way. Into this bare-bones understanding, eugenicists shoehorned a racist and ableist ideology that justified the power of the old American elites.

They argued that because some traits were inherited, that meant some people were inevitably born better: stronger, smarter, perfumed farts, and so on. Those people were the ruling class, but that old order was now supposedly under threat by a rising population of *innately* inferior people—Blacks, Chinese, Irish, Italians, Mexicans, Slavs, Jews, Native Americans, and the Deaf, among many others—who were outbreeding their "natural" betters. The country itself was a body, and minorities, foreigners, people with disabilities, and others were described as diseases infecting it. You probably know the broad outlines because eugenic beliefs were picked up by the Nazis in Germany in the 1930s—they actually consulted with American eugenic organizations and studied American eugenic laws to write their own. :(

Of course, the eugenicist's simplistic view of inheritance, language, and culture was totally wrong—it very much *doesn't work that way*, and their beliefs have been blown out of the water by our modern understanding of genetics, population statistics, and cognitive science.[3] That didn't stop them from scaring a lot of parents, educators, and public officials at the time, and it didn't stop oral advocates from grafting eugenic arguments onto their push for oral education.

In the eugenic model, English was the advanced language of the superior ruling class. ASL, on the other hand, was a primitive, possibly animal-like system—not a real language at all. To the oralist eugenicist, teaching a deaf child to speak English raised them up out of a less-evolved state. This was the modern, scientific, and compassionate thing to do.

While there had been plenty of bigotry toward—and within[4]—the Deaf community before, this was a sinister turn away from older Enlightenment theories about deaf students as rational blank slates. Instead, eugenics explicitly treated deaf people as disease carriers, and deaf schools as unassimilated foreign communities, filled with "defective" people, stubbornly attached to their un-American language and customs. To a group obsessed with breeding, conformity, and disability, this suggested a nightmare scenario: the schools would create a Deaf baby boom that would flood the country with these "inferior" people, crowding out the hearing population. But overturning an already successful and widespread system of deaf education required more than just a philosophy. It needed funding, and it needed a spokesman.

Ring Ring, It's Alec Bell

Alexander Graham Bell was born in Scotland in 1847. He was the child, grandchild, and nephew of elocutionists: teachers of speech and lip-reading for the deaf. He trained and worked as an elocutionist, too. His mother lost her hearing when Bell was twelve, and Bell's wife, Mabel Gardiner Hubbard,

---

[3]Stephen Jay Gould's *The Mismeasure of Man* is a good place to start if you want to learn more about the profound scientific wrongness of eugenics.

[4]From the start, the Deaf community and educators held the same prejudices as the rest of American society. Schools in both the South *and* North were often racially segregated, and students with additional disabilities were often barred from the school, and women were frequently held back from the highest levels of study. Gallaudet, for instance, only graduated its first Black student, the educator Andrew Foster, in 1954.

was also a former student of his; *her* father founded the Clarke School, where Bell taught briefly after moving to the United States, and before moving on to his main passion, invention.

Bell's interest in sound transmission came directly from the family business: he was fascinated by how the body produced and received speech (one of his first experiments was a not-at-all creepy head that said "mama" when you blew into its neck-hole). This eventually led to his invention of the telephone, 1876,[5] which made him enormously wealthy and famous. And despite making his fortune as the founder of Bell Telephone, he continued to advocate for oral education for deaf children for his entire life.

Bell was also an enthusiastic eugenicist; he studied heredity, served on the first eugenic organization in the United States,[6] and helped organize the first International Eugenics Congress. In 1883, he published a hugely influential booklet, *Memoir Upon the Formation of a Deaf Variety of the Human Race*, in which he made the case against sign language-based residential schools from a eugenic perspective:

> Those who believe as I do, that the production of a defective race of human beings would be a great calamity to the world, will examine carefully the causes that lead to the intermarriage of the deaf with the object of applying a remedy.

Bell's recommendations in his *Memoir* were oriented toward reducing the number of deaf babies by assimilating deaf children into the hearing population, encouraging them to find hearing spouses rather than marrying other deaf people. To Bell, that meant enforcing speech and lip-reading, disrupting the generational transmission of ASL as a language, and breaking Deaf culture and the ties that existing deaf schools helped foster.

The plan he laid out in the *Memoir* was straightforward: forbid ASL in deaf schools and move deaf children as much as possible out of a Deaf-majority

---

[5] But ask Elisha Gray and Antonio Meucci how *they* feel. Both these guys *also* invented the telephone, but Bell had better patent lawyers.

[6] The Committee on Eugenics was a subcommittee of the American Breeders' Association—as in *plant breeders*—which focused on human reproduction. Yikes and double yikes.

environment. Their teachers should only be hearing, and as much as possible, they would be encouraged to mix with the hearing population and be isolated from contact with the larger Deaf community. The focus would at all times be on lip-reading and speech, and all instruction would be in English. Oralism should be the law of the land, and sign language would be banned outright.

He succeeded.

1900–1960: Bad New Century

With Bell's enthusiastic public and financial support, both personally and through the AG Bell Foundation, the recommendations of the Milan Conference and the scheme laid out in the *Memoir* were enacted in North America.

By 1900, sign language had been banned in about eighty percent of deaf schools in the United States and Canada. Deaf teachers were fired, and without centers of employment, the Deaf communities around those schools dispersed. Most deaf children were educated in one form of oralism or another, learning only English in the classroom, and had only hearing teachers, never coming into contact with signing Deaf role models. The only hiccup was the schools themselves: while public and private oral day programs were established, many deaf students were still educated in state residential schools.

But if Bell's methods were almost totally adopted, Bell's goals for education and assimilation were an almost total failure. Now-oral residential schools struggled to actually *teach* children—without accessible language, the institutions became warehouses, holding kids until they were adults and turning many of them loose language-deprived, sometimes with only the barest education. Even the children who could manage in oral classrooms were shortchanged because of the time and effort oral methods devoted to speech above other types of learning. As one former student noted, "We spent our entire history class lesson on the French Revolution learning how to pronounce the word 'guillotine.'"

On the other hand, if the goal was to undermine ASL as a language and Deaf culture as a community, Lex Luthor couldn't have done a better job. In a single generation, literacy rates for the Deaf population crashed, and Deaf professionals became a rarity. As the memory of the Deaf Renaissance and its signing celebrities faded, the public's image of successful Deaf adults faded, too. Helped along by eugenic rhetoric, expectations for deaf children dropped away, accelerating the decay of state-supported institutions.

The AG Bell Foundation was enormously successful in imposing its views long after Bell's own death in 1922; not just on education, but in pediatrics and family medicine, and the emerging practices of speech therapy and audiology. Its influence meant that for most of the twentieth century, hearing parents with deaf children were advised by every professional they met to never sign with their children, with the implication that if they did everything just right, their children would learn to speak, lip-read, and be "normal." Sign language was stigmatized, and the AG Bell Foundation campaigned against even the *depiction* of signing Deaf adults in the media. By 1965, most residential schools had essentially given up on academics and were focused on occupational training—according to a government report at the time, there were "no more than a half-dozen true high school programs for the deaf in this country."

The Deaf community saw the catastrophe coming and found some ways to hold on. Deaf social clubs and trade organizations were formed and kept the community informed through meetings and newspapers. The National Association for the Deaf (NAD) got started in 1880, and over the next decades fought a rear-guard battle to preserve ASL and protect deaf schools, along with advocating for the rights of deaf children and adults. Still, the money and the cultural zeitgeist remained with AG Bell and oralism through both World Wars, despite the horrors of the Nazi regime making eugenics itself a dirty word.

Although officially banned from most classrooms, sign language didn't completely vanish. It continued to be used in a few institutions, notably by Gallaudet University and some segregated Black schools in the South, contributing to the emergence of Black American Sign Language as a distinct language. Deaf families as a whole continued to use sign and teach it to their children, and they became important reservoirs of cultural knowledge and history. Sign language was also taught by deaf students to one another and by the few Deaf adults who had contact with them, like residency staff, either openly after school or secretly in the dorms and cafeterias. Still, these efforts were a band-aid on a gaping wound. In the following decades, deaf education remained a dismal affair for most children. Language deprivation was epidemic, and prospects for most deaf kids were dim.

1960–1986: Diamonds and Crap

The first wobble in the dominance of oralism came, ironically, from an English teacher. William Stokoe was a hearing professor of literature at Gallaudet. He wasn't a great signer himself, but he got curious when he saw his students discussing the intricacies of Chaucer in ASL. In 1960, he released *Sign Language Structure*, and in 1965, along with Deaf researchers Carl Cronenburg and Dorothy Casterline, *A Dictionary of American Sign Language on Linguistic Principles*. This was the first time ASL's grammar and syntax had been formally described; recognition that it was a full and sophisticated language was an important step in breaking down the negative stereotypes that had grown up around it.

The next wobble came through the residential schools. Oralism just wasn't effective for most kids, and the gap between what was happening in Deaf homes, where children had access to ASL, and what was happening in oral classrooms was obvious to many educators. In 1967, David Denton, the hearing superintendent for the Maryland School for the Deaf, began to reintroduce sign into the classroom in an ad hoc way and teach sign to the hearing parents of his students. If speech was what worked best for a child, do that. If sign was the most effective tool, use that. The term Total Communication was eventually coined to describe this approach.

The use-as-needed framing helpfully side-stepped some of the old oral versus sign arguments—who could object to something that actually *worked?*—and TC was rapidly adopted by institutions, especially state schools, that could no longer deny oralism's failures. But while this opened the door a crack, the now baked-in bias against ASL and the scarcity of Deaf teachers meant that the impact of TC was less than it could have been. Most TC classrooms ended up staffed by well-meaning hearing educators using a Sim-Com approach with Signed Exact English, another recent "innovation" that left many kids struggling. Still, TC was a crucial but incomplete step toward making language fully accessible to deaf students.

There were other bright spots: in 1969, the National Technical Institute for the Deaf (NTID) was opened at Rochester Institute of Technology, and it quickly expanded into an educational powerhouse. RIT/NTID eventually became the Deaf Yale to Gallaudet's Harvard and encouraged a larger and more diverse class of educated Deaf adults, including Deaf teachers, than any single school could. Cultural institutions like the National Theater for the Deaf, DEAF media, and the Bicultural Center were also founded in the following decade, and awareness of the Deaf community *as a culture* began to re-emerge in the wider public—you might remember Deaf actress Linda Bove as a regular character on Sesame Street starting in 1971.

Legal victories began to give deaf children more educational options as well. *The Rehabilitation Act of 1973* and the *Education for All Handicapped Children Act,* later renamed the *Individuals with Disabilities Education Act* (IDEA) in 1975, were key laws granting access to schools for disabled people and were the result of extraordinary work by disabled activists,[7] including Deaf activists like Dr. Frank Bowe, in support of these laws. Thanks to them, deaf children won the right to a "free and appropriate public education" guided by Individualized Education Plans (IEPs) that held the force of federal law.

But while these laws were a triumph for all disabled Americans, they were a double-edged sword for deaf education. On the one hand, they brought some accountability to residential schools, setting federal standards and legal remedies for neglected institutions, and opening doors for Deaf Disabled students who had been previously shut out. On the other hand, rather than sending your child away to a possibly distant and dilapidated residential institution, deaf children now had the right to attend their presumably better, and hopefully less abusive, local school. Parents could put their deaf children on the same school bus as their hearing siblings and the neighborhood kids, study the same curriculum in the same classes, and have them home for dinner each night.

Sadly, while deaf kids could now *theoretically* receive the same education as their hearing peers, educational approaches for mainstreamed deaf

---

[7]The documentary *Crip Camp* tells this incredible story and gives a lot of context to the legal fights surrounding disability in America that began in the 1970s. Watch it. Watch it. Watch it.

students were still largely tied to oralism or a SimCom, Total Communication method—the same ineffective tactics that were failing kids in the residential schools. Or just as frequently, deaf kids were placed in Special Ed classes that weren't set up for them at all. Regardless of better intentions, this often left children struggling and language-deprived, stranded in hearing classrooms with no peers or role models.

For many oralist educators, this was an unquestioned *good thing*. Mainstreaming meant that the last aspect of Bell's plan from *Memoir* could finally be put in place: placing deaf children in an entirely hearing environment, beyond even the possibility of acquiring sign language or the awareness of a larger Deaf community. While the original motivation for this—preventing more deaf babies—was mostly forgotten, the impulse to assimilate deaf kids into the hearing world at any cost remained strong.

But even for families who didn't think this way, the opportunity to attend a local mainstream school was an exciting experiment. Now that the door was open, sending your deaf child to their local school was a sign of pride, acceptance, and visibility, and the sad conditions of many residential schools made it even more tempting. So even as Deaf teachers and ASL were beginning to creep back into residential school programs, mainstreaming was suddenly pulling deaf kids away from those institutions.

Prosthetic Education

Another major boost for mainstreaming was the advance of modern electronics. Hearing aids, which had been very large and crude prior to the 1960s, started to shrink and become semi-practical to wear on a daily basis. By 1990, cochlear implants started to be available for children as well, allowing some with little to no residual hearing more access to spoken language, too.

While the technology was continually improving, the realities of learning by wire were hard for most hearing professionals to grasp, creating a lot of unfounded confidence about what kids could learn and do using the new devices. Still, more effective hearing prosthetics meant that an ever-more medicalized view of deafness started to dominate professional thinking. Instead of Bell's old notion of using specialized training and education to assimilate deaf children into the hearing world, the view of many professionals shifted to an emphasis on "curing" children. And if a deaf child was cured by technology, then they wouldn't *need* separate schools, or eventually specialized services at all . . .

Oralists adapted by shifting their focus toward the technology, placing a greater emphasis on using hearing aids and implants, and moving away from speechreading and oral training. AG Bell rebranded the old oral education systems as Auditory-Oral Training (AOT) and Auditory-Verbal Training (AVT), under the umbrella term Listening and Spoken Language (LSL)[8] and created a professional licensing system for LSL certification that they controlled, effectively cornering the oral education market. Cochlear implant manufacturers in particular benefited from this shift and aggressively promoted their products to hearing parents and physicians, closely aligning themselves with the rebranded oral education systems and blurring the lines between education and medical treatment. Despite the tactical pivot, many oral schools closed in the 1980s and 1990s under the pressure of mainstreaming, and most of the rest shifted to an early education model, with the idea that kids would move on to mainstream schools after a few years of training to use their devices.

The Deaf community, on the other hand, saw the updated medical model, and CIs in particular, as an existential threat to their heritage and culture, not to mention Yet Another Fucking Thing hearing people were willing to subject deaf children to, rather than just learning to sign. There were passionate arguments and confrontations inside the community and between Deaf activists and CI proponents throughout the 1990s and early 2000s.[9] The CI manufacturers didn't help matters by overselling the effectiveness of their products, or with a series of scandals over defective devices, or with statements like, "The simple fact is that if [Deaf] culture could be reliably wiped out, it would be a good thing to wipe out."[10]

---

[8]A name chosen to suggest equivalence with ASL.

[9]The documentary *The Sound and the Fury* captures this era of the CI debate.

[10]That would be Advanced Bionics CI developer Dr. Michael Merzenich, writing in the *American Psychological Association Monitor* back in 1997.

In the end, because CIs weren't magic and don't transform deaf children into hearing children, the fight over the implants in particular has somewhat receded. Although there are still many folks in the Deaf community and some hearing parents who object to them on principle, these days the focus has shifted away from fights over technology and back to early access to ASL.

Also, in 1984, Prince played a free show at Gallaudet University. What I'm saying is, the period had its ups and downs.

1986–1993: Seven Big Years

In the time between Run-DMC and Wu-Tang Clan, a number of educational and legal events happened in quick succession that profoundly changed the landscape for deaf education. Some were hard to miss, and others were just the seeds of things that have since grown to create the deaf education environment that we see today.

In 1986, Early Intervention was added to the EHA, requiring states to offer services for deaf children from birth to age three and creating the Individualized Family Services Plan (IFSP). This was huge because this meant that states were now required by law to help kids in that tiny window of time *before* the risk of language deprivation set in, possibly preventing the biggest issue in deaf education altogether. In 1990, the law was renamed the *Individuals with Disabilities Education Act* (IDEA), which is how it's now known.

In 1988, dissatisfaction with Total Communication and the resurgent awareness of Deaf culture finally came full circle with the emergence of Bilingual-Bicultural (Bi-Bi) education, an educational philosophy that finally treated ASL as a complete language unto itself, and Deaf culture as a valid identity with its own norms and values. Thanks to the efforts of Deaf educator Marie Jean Philip and others, the Learning Center for the Deaf in Massachusetts, which had been founded as a TC school in 1970, was the first deaf school to fully re-embrace ASL as the language of instruction, abandoning SimCom, sign systems, and other kludges that had taken hold in Total Communication programs.[11]

---

[11] There is a short *documentary, "Bilingual Bicultural Movement" at The Learning Center for the Deaf,* available on YouTube, that's very worth watching.

Despite the advantages that bilingual instruction had, the Bi-Bi model would be a hard sell to many residential schools. The need for fluent ASL signers meant that programs needed time to recruit and retrain staff. Accepting the damage that oralism and Sim-Com / SEE programs had inflicted was a bitter pill for many educators to swallow, so change often hinged on older leadership retiring. Still, Bi-Bi education eventually spread to most of the remaining state schools, empowering Deaf teachers and revitalizing the institutions.

But if changes were happening slowly in residential schools, 1988 was also an earth-shaking year in another part of the Deaf-ed universe: it was the year of Deaf President Now (DPN) at Gallaudet. In 124 years, there had never been a Deaf head of school at Gallaudet University. But in March of '88, the school's board, which was majority hearing, had the choice between three candidates: two Deaf and one hearing. Hopes in the Deaf community ran high that the world's flagship for Deaf education would finally be led by a Deaf educator.

When they chose hearing candidate Elizabeth Zinser, Gallaudet students went HAM. They first marched on the hotel where the trustees were meeting. Then, this being Washington DC, they marched to the Capitol building. The next day, they shut down campus and demanded Zinser resign, and the board move to a majority-Deaf membership. The protesters, led by the "Gallaudet Four"—Greg Hlibok, Jerry Covell, Bridgetta Bourne, and Tim Rarus—were smart, organized, and effective. They made the nightly news for a solid week. Congress got involved. Alumni, teachers, staff, and local interpreters sided with the protesters. The leadership appeared on national TV multiple times, making the case for Deaf self-determination and liberation.

Seven days later, the protesters got everything they asked for. Zinser stepped down, and I. King Jordan, a dean at the school, became the first Deaf president of Gallaudet. Deaf President Now became the landmark event of the modern Deaf rights movement, and its effects rippled out from campus, through the Deaf community and the hearing world. In the wake of DPN, a series of laws was passed to ensure Deaf people more rights and more access to public goods, including the whopper of them all . . .

In 1990, the *Americans with Disabilities Act* (ADA) was signed into law. It is probably the most significant piece of legislation protecting the rights of disabled people in the United States and is almost synonymous with disability law. The ADA was a titanic victory for disability activists and the Deaf community as a whole. It filled in many of the cracks left by the *Rehabilitation Act* and IDEA, encompassing state services, private schools and colleges, businesses, and other places not receiving federal funds. This has an enormous effect on deaf adults, finally requiring virtually all public venues to accommodate them, making new careers and opportunities available. This was very, very good, but the ADA's impact on pre-K and elementary education wasn't as pronounced—IDEA and the *Rehabilitation Act* had already done most of the heavy lifting in public schools. If you're looking for something that has a direct impact on deaf *children*, another event happens three years later that might be even more important.

In 1993, the National Institutes of Health Consensus Development Conference on Early Identification of Hearing Impairment convened to issue a set of recommendations for childhood hearing. The most important of which was simple: screen all infants' hearing within three months of birth. This was the work of audiologist Marion Downs, who had advocated for universal infant screening for decades. With modern technology like ABR, newborns could have basic hearing tests done before they came home from the hospital and *before* the risk of language deprivation set in. This changed the game. In 1993, fewer than ten percent of newborns were screened for deafness in the United States. By 2018, about ninety-five percent were.

1993–today: Learning in the Aftermath

So by the mid-1990s, all the pieces seemed to be in place for a second Deaf Renaissance: early identification, early intervention, strong educational rights, access to ASL in (some) schools, not to mention ever-improving hearing technology. Science began to catch up, too—a growing group of hearing and Deaf researchers began teasing out the effects of early language access and early language deprivation in deaf children, with both population studies and previously impossible MRI imaging that showed the structural impact that access to language had on developing brains.

And yet . . . the "deaf achievement gap" is still with us. Deaf kids have remained starkly underserved by school districts to this day, and this is reflected in an ongoing epidemic of language deprivation and overall awful academic performance in almost every area. Although the research and resources were out there, the way the law was structured meant that parents often weren't given sufficient information on early language acquisition, and local Early Intervention didn't have to conform to any particular standards when assisting families with deaf children. And mostly, their standards still sucked.

In 2010, Deaf activist Sheri Ann Farinha founded the LEAD-K movement to address the gap. The point of LEAD-K was to require states to actually track the progress of deaf children in the Early Intervention system from birth and set statewide expectations for early language acquisition that can then be enforced through the IFSP / IEP system.

In 2015, California became the first state to pass LEAD-K, despite the initial opposition of AG Bell and the American Speech-Language-Hearing Association (ASHA). In 2019, LEAD-K brought AG Bell's national organization to the table, and they agreed to settle their differences in order to make headway on the continuing problem of deaf student underachievement; although collaborating with "the enemy" was sharply controversial in both the Deaf and oralist educational communities, small changes to the bill were agreed upon, and AG Bell dropped their opposition. As of this writing, there are nineteen states[12] with LEAD-K laws on the books and more campaigns ongoing.

But new developments in special education are ominous. As of 2025, President Trump has made sustained efforts to defund and disband the Department of Education, which disburses funds to both Gallaudet and NTID, as well as oversees enforcement of IDEA and Section 504. Additionally, there has been a major legal assault on Section 504 by conservative state attorneys general, attempting to have it declared unconstitutional. How this will play out at the district level remains to be seen, but parents will need to be vigilant and politically active in order to keep their children safe.

---

[12]Oregon, California, Nevada, Arizona, Montana, South Dakota, Nebraska, Kansas, Texas, Louisiana, Michigan, Indiana, Georgia, South Carolina, Virginia, West Virginia, Maine, New Jersey, Connecticut

History, What the Shit?

Today, deaf education is under assault. There are vital and effective deaf programs in many states, but the vast majority of deaf children receive inadequate and half-baked educations in mainstream settings. For every new bilingual school or program that opens, state legislators move to shut down historic institutions as political stunts or as collateral damage from budget cuts. Massachusetts has four bilingual deaf schools within its borders. Neighboring Vermont has none. Eugenics is back on the rise in the MAGA movement, ready to cut funds and saddle deaf students with low expectations and substandard teaching. It's not fair to our children, and it's not fair to us, the parents. But this is the starting point, and knowing where things stand gives you a chance to get your child everything they need.

What's the Deal with Natural Languages, and What's the Problem with Sign Systems?

I mentioned in the first chapter that the deaf educational world is crawling with schemes that look like sign language but which aren't natural languages at all. These are the sign systems: a mess of methods that have been offered over the years as substitutes for American Sign Language. Most of them didn't start out as NutraSweet ASL but were invented for other specific educational purposes, like teaching English literacy or speech therapy. But since all of them are easier for hearing teachers to learn—let's face it, checkers is easier than chess—and most of them *seem* like spoken English, they started to sneak into general deaf education and be offered as L1s to babies. These days, you are more likely to meet hearing educators using one of these sign systems than you are using ASL, but **compared with an accessible natural language, no sign system is a good choice as an L1 for deaf children.**

The basic problem is that sign systems take the modality of sign,[13] and back it up with language that's either half-baked, broken, or just can't be fluently

---

[13] Modality is the method by which you express a language—signing, speaking, typing, whistling, and so on.

expressed in that modality. At best, learning a sign system is more like learning to read and write, not a language itself but a secondary skill that you need a language to master in the first place. At worst, they're like trying to sing an opera in Morse code. Not only is this at odds with how children actually learn, but it also explains why the problems with sign systems are so difficult for educators to spot. Because they *represent* English in one form or another, an adult who already understands English can muddle through with a sign system, while denying the fundamental experience of learning a fluent first language to a deaf child.

This can be a confusing topic: teachers and other professionals don't always know, or can't always explain this fundamental difference between a natural language and a sign system. It's just not very straightforward, especially when you've got to unpack loaded terms like "natural."

Natural Languages

In linguistics, a *natural language* is any signed or spoken language that grows, unplanned, in a community of people. As far as we know, natural languages are innate to human society—they develop through human interaction on a generational scale. There are language-deprived people, but there are no language-deprived cultures. And although they are incredibly diverse, natural languages all have some kind of regular grammar and syntax, and they're all able to express the full range of human ideas and emotions, from dad jokes to driver's ed courses to pillow talk. English, Estonian, and ASL are all natural languages. Dothraki, JavaScript, and Furbish are not.

Beyond their surface differences, we have evidence that natural languages share a set of subtle traits that make them easy for babies to learn and then to think with. We also have evidence that artificial sign systems lack these traits—their "language-ness" is somehow disrupted or incomplete. These missing traits aren't always obvious or even completely known, but they make the difference between a child who has full access to their potential and one who's been limited by the neurological trauma of language deprivation.

Neat Is Not Natural

One aspect of "naturalness" that's a little hard to wrap your mind around is how *messy* it really is. Because they're rooted in our incredibly complex brains and constantly being reshaped through millions of interactions on a daily basis among thousands of people, natural languages are many times more sophisticated than any artificial communication system could possibly be.

Sign systems are often presented as attempts to "fix" messiness and make things easy, but this gets it exactly backwards. Children don't need simplification—they need complexity, because thinking is complex. Any scheme that professionals have come up with pales in comparison to the natural processes of language acquisition that have been in place in children's brains for thousands of years.

Imagine a chaotic patch of jungle and a tidy backyard garden. Compared with the garden, a jungle might seem like an intimidating place, but that's because it's so much more varied and fertile. Your garden can only give you the things you put there yourself; you plant tomatoes and you get tomatoes. But what if you unexpectedly need a mango, or a poisonous berry, or a jaguar? Compared with man-made systems, natural language gives our kids an almost limitless variety of things to think and to say.

Don't give your kid tomatoes, give them jaguars.

Signed Exact English and Friends

There arean array of different sign English systems floating around, including Signed Exact English (SEE), Sign English (SE), Sign Supported English (SSE), Manually Coded English (MCE), and Conceptually Accurate Signed English (CASE).

SEE and its offshoots are more or less word-for-word transpositions of English into a sign system that takes most of its vocabulary from ASL. But unlike ASL, SEE has articles like "a" and "the," prefixes and suffixes like "pre-" and "-ing," and other modifications to make its grammar and syntax match English. Hearing teachers like to present these systems to parents as a good middle ground between ASL and spoken English, just like a hotdog milkshake is a good middle ground between dinner and dessert.

SEE started life in the mid-1960s as a teaching tool to help Deaf kids with their literacy—a specialized system that could help teach written English in a visual way. That didn't work, but because of the ingrained bias against ASL that was common at the time, SEE metastasized across deaf education as a *substitute* for ASL. These days, SEE is the most common sign system in the United States and Canada, especially in Total Communication programs, where it's offered as an L1 to thousands of infants and toddlers. Because of this, it does an enormous amount of harm.

These systems have gone through several revisions and remakes, but they all suffer the same general problems:

SimCom blues: Because SEE matches English structure, it's everybody's favorite sign system to SimCom. But hearing SEE signers do to SEE what they do to ASL when they SimCom—they drop signs and mangle the grammar without realizing it, because their fluency in spoken English makes it easy to overlook the mistakes on their hands. SimCom is still not easy, though, and teachers end up simplifying their *spoken* English so their signs can keep up, so kids who have access to speech get a watered-down version of English on top of everything else.

SEE-low: It also turns out that your hands are just slower than your mouth. Obvious joke aside, this means that you can't cram all of spoken English into a sign system and keep up a regular conversational pace. A skillful SEE signer—or even an ASL signer—can only produce about one sign for every three words an English speaker can voice. This is a big deal; fluency is partly a measure of how quickly you get your ideas out.

Because of this, ASL has developed a different grammar than English, a spatial grammar, where the area around your body, along with your gaze, expressions, and posture adds detail and structure to sentences. This helps to speed up and clarify the language. So while English uses more words per minute than ASL, they both express *ideas* at about the same rate.[14]

But SEE lacks spatial grammar; it doesn't exist in English so it *can't* exist in SEE. Going back to Christine Sun Kim's piano metaphor, if spoken English is like playing a one-handed melody, and ASL is like playing two-handed chords,

---

[14]In computer lingo, English has a faster write speed, but ASL has better data compression.

a SEE signer is picking out notes with just one *finger*. Halting or very slow expression doesn't adequately model fluent language for deaf children, and it has a big impact on the ability of children to decode the English grammar that they are supposed to acquire from SEE. Even when done properly, SEE becomes long chains of signs that need to be "read" meticulously, a skill kids without a strong first language can't manage. When signed in a quick-and-dirty fashion, SEE becomes a less-than-a-language mush where grammar and conceptual correctness fall by the wayside.

Conceptual inaccuracy: SEE's lack of language-ness is most obvious when you look at its vocabulary. When SEE was created, English homophones were directly transferred into SEE vocabulary in an arbitrary way, so the word "butterfly" was initially expressed in the ASL signs for BUTTER—like the delicious grease—and FLY—like what a bird do. Because of this, SEE is a patchwork of lookalike signs, which stand for things that have no relationship to one another.

In newer forms of SEE, that's been cleaned up to a degree, but it still exists: for example, in English, the word "park" can mean "the thing you do with your car" or "the place with a lot of grass and trees." The problem is that the makers of SEE used only one sign for both meanings, and it's literally ASL for "park a car," which includes the handshape used to describe automobiles. Kids who have SEE as their L1 end up struggling through a language that has somehow conceptually linked these two ideas arbitrarily because of their sound in a language they can't hear.

This sort of thing actually happens all the time in natural languages, too—there are tons of homophones and weird word borrowing in spoken English *and* in ASL—but natural language structures provide subtle hints that tell children how to learn and use them, which helps support the underlying meaning. But in a slow and grammatically impoverished system like SEE, those structures are absent or incomplete.

All this comes out in a notable symptom for some kids who've gotten SEE as a substitute for a language: a tendency to struggle with abstract reasoning skills. But those struggles, which are the hallmark of language deprivation, are hard to spot in infants and toddlers. Kids can end up far down a road, being able to use SEE signs for basic communication, but getting stuck developmentally because they don't pick up the underlying cognitive scaffolding that natural languages provide.

Lack of community support: The last flaw for SEE is that it's not used much outside of schools. Some pre-K programs will actually explicitly state this: "We use SEE here—the kids transition to ASL when they go to the deaf school." Ignoring the fact that SEE is going to set them back in their language skills, possibly forever, this means that teaching kids SEE strands them: there are few SEE interpreters in the world, not much media in SEE, and generally just not much post-graduation, or even post-elementary, available for a SEE user. The adult Deaf community operates in ASL and that's where the resources, energy, and people are.

SEE is disliked by many in the Deaf community, either because they were subjected to it growing up or because they see it, rightly, as stealing from ASL while sidelining actual Deaf language and culture. Some of the most spectacular online arguments happen when folks are debating whether a given sign is "really" ASL or was slipped back into the language from SEE. But purity politics aside, SEE, at best, gives deaf kids a lot to unlearn as they get older—it's an anti-education. Avoid it if you can.

Pidgin Signed English (PSE and Contact Sign)

PSE didn't start as a sign system, but more as an observation: starting in the late 1960s, language researchers noticed that in environments with both English and ASL speakers, some fluent signers used their ASL in a more Englishy way, and less-fluent signers mixed English grammar into ASL inconsistently. This was initially called "contact sign"—the signing that was used where the Deaf and hearing communities were in contact. It was later relabeled Pidgin Sign English, "pidgin" meaning a communication system that merges two or more languages without having regular grammar or syntax.

The idea of PSE eventually entered the general consciousness, so these days, some folks will say "I sign more PSE" to indicate that their ASL is still beginner-intermediate level. That's not a huge problem itself; especially if you're a hearing parent, there's no shame in not having perfect ASL. You probably started learning as an adult, under the shittiest circumstances. *You* don't need seamless, error-free ASL to raise a deaf kid with strong language skills, but your kid does need exposure to fluent ASL somewhere. If that somewhere isn't at home *and* it isn't at school, your child is more likely to get hit with the language deprivation stick.

Low standards are no standards: PSE becomes a problem when it's promoted by hearing educators as an end goal for you or your child, or as a language of instruction in the classroom. Don't let that three-letter acronym fool you—it's not ASL with training wheels on, it's just *incorrect and inconsistent* ASL. The PSE brand name does nothing but give poor language skills a shiny label and legitimacy they don't deserve.

Any time hearing teachers start pushing PSE on you, you know a couple of things: they can't function as language models for your children, they probably don't have a strong grasp of childhood language acquisition to begin with, and their program couldn't be bothered to hire qualified Deaf adults or other fluent signers. None of these are good things. And if you're a beginning or intermediate signer, it's better not to use PSE as a description of your signing; just say, "I'm a beginner" or "I'm working on my ASL," and leave it there. Avoid anyone who wants to teach you PSE—there's no reason on God's green earth that you should waste time with anything but a real language, either.

Note that there are ways ASL and English *do* mix fluently; ASL is a minority language in an English-speaking country, so skillful bilingual speakers will naturally pick up words, phrases, and constructions from English to use in ASL; they might also speak or write English in more ASL-like ways, too! This *code-switching* is a sign of fluency and adds layers of expression to both languages. But those are advanced skills for people with mastery of both languages—the opposite of what's happening with PSE.

Cued Speech (CS, Cueing, Cued English)

Cueing is a phonetic representation of English, stringing a small number of handshapes together on the face and mouth to visually sound out whole words and sentences like the stenography of a court reporter. It was initially developed as a speech-teaching tool for deaf kids and a way to make the various sounds of the English language visible to children who couldn't hear them. Like SEE, it's been around since the 1960s, but it's less popular. It's closely associated with an English literacy program for deaf kids called Visual Phonics, and sometimes used as a supplement in either ASL, SEE, or oral environments, and it even has its proponents in the Deaf community as a reading and pronunciation tool.

The problem comes when Cued Speech gets offered to hearing families as a first language for their kids. Because it's based on English and only uses a few handshapes, it's promoted as faster and easier for parents to learn. This is fine as far as it goes, but it doesn't take you very far. Because it's transposing English into a non-native modality, Cued Speech has many of the drawbacks of SEE: it was never intended to be an L1, and it doesn't give kids the full natural language experience—again, it's akin to teaching a baby to read before they can talk.

There's a relatively small group of professionals and families that use it, and only a few institutions across the country have it in the curriculum, but teaching CS as a first language is kind of like teaching Hooked On Phonics as an L1: you're using pantyhose to strain spaghetti, and the spaghetti is your kid's brain.

Sign Supported English (SSE)

Although it has a different meaning in the United Kingdom (where it's a form of signed English like SEE), in the United States, Sign Supported English can mean a kind of SimCom lite: speaking English sentences with main words or new concepts being represented with signs from ASL.

Like PSE, you might find yourself doing this at certain points if you're using spoken language with your kid. You talk until you come across a word that's new or one that needs clarification, then sign the word to explain it or make it more comprehensible, preferably separating the languages using the "sandwich" of talk /SIGN / talk or SIGN / talk / SIGN. Using one language to support the development of another is a totally kosher tactic, part of a larger set of learning strategies known as *translanguaging*.

But if a deaf child's hearing levels are such that they need their spoken language spiked with sign, that's an indication that their first language should be entirely visual—spoken language isn't fully accessible to them, and that's what you need for robust cognitive development. As one wrench in the toolbox, it's fine, but as an L1, it'll get you in trouble.

Makaton

Makaton isn't really *a thing* here in the United States, but it bears mentioning because it's big in the United Kingdom and well-known because it's used in the children's show *Something Special*. Makaton was initially designed in Britain to communicate with people with motor or developmental disabilities that prevented their use of spoken language. You can see where this is going; British Sign Language got chopped up and used in a piecemeal and non-grammatical way, and once it caught on with special educators, they tried inflicting it on deaf kids. Don't get bamboozled. Makaton is not a language and not a good L1 option for your deaf child.

What's the Deal with Augmentative and Alternative Communication (AAC)?

AAC is the umbrella term for tools some people with disabilities might use to get their point across if spoken or signed language isn't available to them. The classic AAC is a picture board a person can point to in order to ask for specific things or express feelings or thoughts, but it really covers a range of tools from simple gestures all the way to sophisticated apps and speech synthesizers like the one Stephen Hawking was famous for.

AAC can be an enormous support for some kids, and when used as part of speech-language therapy, AAC can help children get their needs met and also help with explicit language acquisition in both ASL and English. Deaf disabled kids, in particular might use AAC if they have a motor or communication disability that interferes with their expressive speech or signing. However, AAC is not a language and should not be used as a substitute for deaf kids in place of a signed language. **Deaf kids who use AAC because of other disabilities also need exposure to ASL in order to build their receptive language skills and scaffold their cognitive abilities.**

Be especially wary of any SLP or other professional who suggests your child should use AAC in place of ASL because it's "too hard" for them or their teachers / caregivers to learn. While it will ease communication, it's a far cry from a natural language, and it won't prevent language deprivation on its own. Also, be wary of any professional who labels ASL *as an AAC*. ASL is a language, one of the languages your child might use. Defining it as an alternative to language shows that the pro in question might have some serious biases under their belt.

Early Intervention, Special Education, and IDEA

When we signed up for Early Intervention, the district sent us a huge stack of pamphlets: Please Don't Sue Us, Here's How Not to Sue Us, Here's What You Can Do Instead of Suing Us, etc.
So that was useful.

my wife

In the United States, services for families of deaf babies ages 0–3 are delivered through a process called Early Intervention (EI). EI programs go by different titles depending on the state: Early Start, Help Me Grow, Baby Watch, and so on. Whatever alarming name they give it, this is the system that gets your child things like special preschool classes, speech-language pathology, and other services to help them and your family be as successful as possible. This is important because unless you are a kajillionaire, you'll want the government to help pay for it all—and most public programs for deaf kids aren't accessible without a referral from EI.

Deaf and hard of hearing kids generally qualify for Early Intervention as long as they have a medical diagnosis of "hearing loss" that fits your state's definition for deaf, hearing impaired, or deafblind. Families should get referred to EI from a doctor, audiologist, or other professional as soon as the diagnosis is confirmed, but if for some reason that didn't happen, you can also register your family by contacting your state EI offices—just Google "Early Intervention self-referral <your state>."

EI services are managed by different local government organizations depending on where you live. It's sometimes your school district, but it can also be a multi-district agency or other entity. These are referred to as the Local Educational Agency (LEA[15]). Once your child leaves EI, they are then picked up by the local Special Education (SpEd) provider, which again can be the local school district, regional body, or other organization. There's no gap in coverage, and that entity will be providing services until your child is age twenty-one.

It's important to know that even though the details vary state-to-state and community-to-community, Early Intervention and Special Education are governed by a federal law, the *Individuals with Disabilities Education Act* (IDEA).[16] This requires states to offer EI and SpEd services via IDEA, then the states use different schemes to administer these services to kids. What this ultimately means is that if you have a problem with how your district is treating you and your child, knowing what your rights are under IDEA is your best shot at getting what you need. The law is not perfect, and the Trump administration is taking steps to undermine its enforcement, but it remains the law of the land.

Note that Early Intervention and Special Education isn't *just* for deafness. IDEA covers a vast range of disabilities,[17] and your state is required to provide all the services your kid needs to succeed right from the start.

IEP, IFSP, 504, WTF?

These are the names for the three common types of educational / therapeutic intervention plans used for deaf children under US law, and the three-word phrase you will often speak in conjunction with them. They are the master

---

[15]Confusingly, LEA representatives are also called LEAs. So in this book, I mostly refer to LEA organizations as "the district" and their rep as "the LEA."

[16]While IDEA is the primary law that covers early intervention and special education services in the United States, there are two other major laws that play a role in the education of deaf children: the *Rehabilitation Act of 1973* and *the Americans with Disabilities Act* (ADA).

[17]The official list as of 2023: Autism, Deaf-blindness, Deafness, Emotional Disturbance, Hearing Impairment, Intellectual Disabilities, Multiple Disabilities, Orthopedic impairment, Other Health Impairment (OHI), Specific learning disability, Speech or language impairment, Traumatic brain injury, and Visual impairment including blindness.

plans for which services or accommodations are given to your child through the local school district, and they start coming together as soon as your district knows you have a deaf kid. You will be talking about these things with other parents, you will post memes about your plans, you will dream about them. To have a deaf kid is to have an IFSP, IEP, or 504.

Individual Family Service Plans (IFSPs) manage all services for your baby and your family from birth to age three. Every deaf baby should have one—the whole point of Early Intervention is to get a kid an IFSP and started with services before they get to school age.

Individual Educational Plans (IEPs) take over after an IFSP is done, age three to twenty-one. They are similar to IFSPs but focused entirely on the kid, with no services for the family. If your child is over the age of three when they're identified as deaf, you should start with an IEP.

504 plans are alternatives to IFSPs and IEPs that are a holdover from an older, less stringent federal law, Section 504 of the *Rehabilitation Act of 1973*. They determine accommodations that are offered through your local school, but don't provide for outside services, don't have as much oversight, and have fewer routes for appeal when the district isn't coming through. Compared to IEPs, 504s are hot garbage on a crispy cracker and should be avoided if possible.

IFSP / IEP meetings are where these plans are created. They can be crowded: they include you, your spouse or partner if you have one, and any other caregivers you want to attend. They also include your kid's treatment team—whatever speech-language pathologists, physical or occupational therapists, teachers of the deaf, and other professionals work with them on language acquisition or other areas relevant to school, as well as the district's representative, the LEA.

In theory, meetings should be happy and relaxed affairs where everyone celebrates your kid's progress and makes plans for their ongoing success. In reality, they're often tense and mostly awful. While you're there to get the best services for your child, the district's interests are usually focused on saving money and not provoking a lawsuit. This means the LEA will often not be very forthcoming about what they could be giving your child, and not very enthusiastic when you present your ideas. If you have disagreements with them or your kid's team about what your child needs, they can be nightmarish.

The keys to survival are picking and preparing your team, making your decisions before you go to the meeting, and understanding your rights as a parent. **Your local Deaf services agency, Hands and Voices chapter, as well as Language First, the American Society for Deaf Children (ASDC), and other advocacy organizations can provide training on IFSPs, IEPs, and 504s for parents to help you get a handle on this process. They will have tutorials and seminars that go far beyond the information in this book, and I highly suggest doing additional research.**

Even better is finding a Deaf educational advocate to help make your plans and attend meetings with you. You may find advocates at your local deaf services agency, your local school, through the ASDC, or hire them privately. If you can get one, they are worth their fucking weight in gold.

504 meetings are typically much smaller. Depending on your state regulations, they can be just your child's classroom teacher and other pros or representatives from the school itself. Federal law gives no specific requirements for who must be there—not even the parents—which is one reason why 504s are not a great option.

IFSP and IEP Quick Start Guide

Although they have important differences, you're going to use the same strategies to get through IFSP and IEP meetings. It is a very bureaucratic process; if you can find trusted advisors who know the law to help you navigate these meetings, that's the biggest help of all. But since you've probably got a baby in your lap right now and a meeting already on the calendar, here are my essential tips.

An IFSP or IEP is a legally binding contract between you and your school district. Whatever is written in the document is basically the *entire commitment your district has to assist and educate you and your child.* If something's written in the plan, the district has a legal obligation to recognize it and make it happen. If it's not in the plan, it doesn't exist. Get it all on paper.

You can call an IFSP or IEP meeting at any time. If you need to add a new service or are not receiving a service written in the plan, or need to make other changes, you can call a new meeting with your LEA. You don't have to wait for the next six-month (IFSP) or yearly (IEP) scheduled meeting.

IFSPs and IEPs have three critical parts:

1. **Assessments** are any measurements or descriptions of your child's cognitive, linguistic, physical, and social-emotional development. These can either be written observations by you, other caregivers, or teachers and professionals, or they can be school grades or formal tests with names like the *Hawaii Early Learning Profile* or the *ASL Communication Development Inventory.*
2. **Goals** are targets that you and your team set for your child's learning and development. Goals have to be written in a very specific way to make sure they can be measured, recorded, and met.
3. **Services** are all the various classes and therapies your child (and your family, for IFSPs) will receive from the district, including special preschool enrollment, ASL lessons, or appointments with a speech-language pathologist, as well as in-school accommodations and modifications, to help reach those goals.

The three parts work in a cycle:

1. Assessments look at your child's abilities and help set the goals you want them to reach.
2. Goals determine which services your child receives for the next six or twelve months.
3. Services support your child's learning and development over that period, trying to reach those goals.
4. New assessments given at the end of the six or twelve-month period determine whether your kid has met the goals and determine the *next* set of goals for the next IFSP / IEP.

'Round and around it goes.

Since IFSPs and IEPs are essentially asking, "Who pays for that?", go into your meetings with a contract-negotiation mindset. Not a "let's see if we can come to an agreement," kind of negotiation, but more of a "we're from the union and here are our demands," thing. School districts are notorious for guiding parents away from more expensive services in general. If they're hostile to ASL, they'll go to great lengths to block access to sign language services and talk enormous shit about the local deaf school, and they will apply a lot of pressure to get their way. Ask me how I know.

Always make sure you understand what services are being delivered, and what your goals are, and get clarification if you're confused about *anything*. If you see something in the documents you don't agree with, make sure it's corrected with language that you approve. Never sign a plan if there's something in it that you don't understand or don't like.

The IFSP tells a story about where your child will eventually go to school. If you're aiming for placement at a specific program, mention it by name, emphasize those goals and services that fit into the program's philosophy, and express your own desires early and get them written into the assessments. This will then set the tone for the transition to an IEP, which is when pre-K and elementary school choices will start being made. For instance, if you want to place your kid in a bilingual-bicultural school, make sure you include both ASL and English in your goals, and use the words "bilingual" and "bilingual-bicultural" in your descriptions of goals and services, and talk about aiming for a specific program in the future.

We had a number of unpleasant fights around our kid's IFSP, always centered on us wanting our kid to have *both* English and ASL services. It sucked balls, but when we finally got to the IEP transition meeting and asked for placement at our excellent local deaf school, we didn't get a peep of protest from the district. We'd planted those seeds already.

IFSPs and IEPs are *individual*. You don't have to settle for what your home district offers you. Don't be shy about shopping around to different programs or professionals outside your district and cobbling together or ordering "off-menu"—plans are supposed to allow things like split placement between two programs or school districts, using multiple languages or approaches for a given issue, or bringing in third-party services if the district doesn't offer them. Different districts may have restrictions or say they have restrictions on this, but in reality, the law gives parents a lot of leeway to insist on getting the services they ask for.

IFSPs are for the whole family. IEPs are for your child *only*. If you need services for yourself or the rest of the family so you can support your child—things like sign language classes, or Deaf mentors for hearing siblings, or respite care funds so you can get a break from watching your child, the district may pay for them until your child turns three. Once your child is three and has moved over to an IEP, the district will only pay for services that go directly to your kid.

Things to Do Before Your IFSP / IEP Meeting

Build your team. You don't have the time or energy to fight with professionals who undermine your decisions. Figure out which of the SLPs, ToDs, and other pros in your child's orbit you trust and who support you. They're your squad. Sideline everyone else. See "Firing your Pros" for more on this.

Get a Deaf educational advocate if you can. An educational advocate can attend meetings with you, cite state and federal regulations chapter and verse, and bake a big batch of IDEA biscuits for administrators if they aren't following the law. Having a Deaf professional at the table also immediately changes the tone of the meeting—administrators are a lot more reluctant to say bullshit like, "you have to choose between ASL and English" in front of them. Your local deaf school's outreach center, or your local deaf services agency is the first place to look for free help, but you can also find them in private practice or at other disability rights agencies, too.

When we were having issues with our district, we got an advocate from our deaf services agency. They sent us a petite Deaf lawyer at no cost to us, but we might as well have brought a live panther to the meeting—we suddenly got a *lot* of respect, and with her help, we were able to properly assert our rights as parents.

You can bring (almost) anyone you want to an IFSP or IEP meeting, as long as they can testify to the well-being and educational / therapeutic needs of your child. In addition to an educational advocate, you can bring family members or other caregivers, Deaf relatives, a Deaf mentor, an outside SLP, a neuropsychologist, or other professional, although you may have to pay pros for their time.[18] Numbers matter; the more folks on your side in the IFSP / IEP meeting, the more likely you are to get your way.

You can exclude (almost) anyone you want from an IFSP or IEP meeting. This is the flipside of building your team. That SLP who doesn't know shit about pediatric deafness? Request that they not attend the meeting, but instead submit a written report two weeks in advance.[19] Then read it and share it with your friendly professionals, and be ready to reply in the meeting with only your people and the LEA present. You may also have the right to meet with regional district officials—the boss's boss—rather than the LEA if you need to (it varies by state). In general, IFSP and IEP meetings are *your* space.

You can demand assessments for your child from *any* qualified professional. This means that if the district has your child tested by an SLP or other professional with no background in deaf children, or who otherwise gives you the heebie-jeebies, you can request assessment from a deaf-savvy, or even better, a Deaf professional. You *always* have the right to a second opinion for assessments, and the district has to pay for the assessment unless they want to challenge your request in an administrative motion, which they're not likely to do. Language First maintains a list of deaf-savvy, pro-ASL SLPs and other professionals on their website—it's a good place to start if you need to find competent assessors.

Make your decisions before the meeting. If you have a spouse or partner, make sure you're on the same page, and plan ahead with them and your chosen team members. Decide in advance what your goals are, which assessors or assessments you want, and what services you're asking for. Keep a list handy during the meeting and check items off as they're addressed. It always helps to write down specific things you want in the plan—you can literally just staple it to the IEP / IFSP if you need to, and it becomes part of the contract.

---

[18]You'll need to send a notification in writing to the IFSP / IEP team, including the person's name and role:

"Jane Motherbear, caregiver, will be attending the IEP meeting on June 2."

[19]You'll also need to send a written request about this: "John Smallberries, SLP, will not attend the meeting on June 2. He will submit a written report at least two weeks in advance."

Don't wait until you're sitting down with the team to figure it out—it's absolutely the worst time to make decisions. Every once in a while someone from the district will suggest something helpful that you haven't anticipated, but for the most part, you set the agenda.

Setting goals is important. Don't let administrators or bad professionals lowball you on goals. Low expectations for deaf kids, especially deaf kids with additional disabilities, are epidemic, but they're a lot cheaper and easier for school districts to meet. Check if your state has passed a LEAD-K law—they contain strong developmental goals for deaf infants and children. If your state *doesn't* have LEAD-K, the milestones from California's LEAD-K bill, SB210, make great goals, and you don't need to live in California to use them for your child; they're linked from my website, willfertman.com, but you can just google them. For our kid's plan, we printed out and attached SB210 milestones to his IFSP and wrote that "in addition to whatever other goals we set, we're also using SB210."

Also, keep in mind that you can set as many goals as you need to, to make sure that each of your educational and developmental concerns is addressed. Again, this is especially important for Deaf + or Deaf Disabled kids.

IEPs need all goals framed in a "deficit model." Unlike IFSPs, IEPs only cover services that address your child's academic weaknesses—areas where they are measurably below average. This is a problem for deaf kids because some districts will yank needed services, up to and including classroom interpreters, if a kid is doing well. *This cuts out the supports that were allowing them to succeed in the first place.* Carefully setting goals and talking about how your child still lags in areas, whether you believe it or not, allows you to stay inside that deficit model while your child continues to get what they need to do well. This can be tricky, but deaf-ed advocates and deaf-savvy professionals are familiar with this challenge and can be valuable guides.

Make separate goals for each language. If you plan on teaching your child English and ASL, or any other combination of languages, all the language goals on the IFSP or IEP should have separate entries. Because goals drive services, if your goal is "My child will have a vocabulary of 20 words by 18 months," the district has an excuse not to offer ASL services; the goal is to teach twenty words—you didn't specify *which* language, and the default is always English.

Instead, each language gets its own goal: "My kid will have a vocabulary of 20 words in ASL by 18 months" *and* "My kid will have a vocabulary of 20 words in English at 18 months." They are then obligated to offer services that will help do both those things. As they grow, their ASL and English assessments will change, so their goals for each language will end up different—that's fine, just don't merge them together.

Separate speech and hearing goals from expressive and receptive *language* goals. A bad plan will have a lot of picky shit in it about your kid making certain sounds with their mouth, or hearing particular noises in the speech range—the Ling 6 sounds in particular—but little in it about *understanding* words and being able to express needs via complex language. Speech is not language, and hearing is not understanding. Focusing too much on speech is a recipe for language deprivation.

It's ok to have speech goals, but there should always be more functional language goals than speech production or sound reception goals in the plan: "my kid will point to the animal named in ASL" or "my kid will respond appropriately to the word 'no' in English," rather than "my kid will correctly pronounce the 't' sound" or "my kid will hear the difference between 's' and 'sh' sounds." And always make separate goals for receptive and expressive language in each of the languages you want your child to learn.

Preview your decisions with the participants beforehand. A week or two before your scheduled meeting, send around a list of your goals for your kid and an outline of services you'll be asking for to everyone who will attend the meeting. Bureaucrats don't like surprises, and it saves huge amounts of time if you don't need to sit there and recite every assessment and goal at the start of the meeting. Even if you're asking for things they won't necessarily agree to, it opens the door to the district finding a way to accommodate you. It also gives your team a chance to prepare and defend your decisions.

At the Meeting

Ask people to state their experience and credentials in their introductions. If you've found your squad and have experienced professionals, especially Deaf professionals, ready to contribute, it's a good way to emphasize who the experts are in the room.

Identify who the LEA is at the start of the meeting. In every meeting, there will be one person, selected by the district, who represents the district, knows what services the district offers, and can approve IFSP and IEP expenses. Every IFSP and IEP meeting must have an LEA present, and all questions about what services the district will supply should be directed to them, as they are the only ones in the meeting with the power to determine what money gets spent on your child. If they don't have a yes or no answer right away, they are obligated to give you an answer within ten business days following the meeting.

You can call "time out." If a meeting seems to be going off the rails, or if you need a few minutes to talk with your partner, your advocate, or another professional at the meeting, you can pause, go to a private place or mute the Zoom call, and talk over your options. Bad school districts will try to hustle you through a meeting; don't let them.

You *never* need to approve an IFSP or IEP plan. One of the biggest tricks districts play is giving parents the impression that you need to sign an IFSP or IEP in order to end the meeting, or that the meeting is all the time you will ever have to set the plan. If you feel like you need more time, you can leave the meeting without signing the plan, take it home and read it, and consult with your partner and your professional team. Then, if you need to, you can suggest changes via email or in a second meeting—only sign the plan when you're satisfied with what's in it. *The district must continue the services it was providing before until you agree on the contents of a new IFSP or IEP.*

You can stop a meeting at any time. If you feel like a meeting isn't going well, or you can't come to an agreement with the district, you can hit the bricks and come back later with reinforcements. Just tell the group that you're ending the meeting and that you'll contact the LEA to reschedule. Administrators hate IFSP and IEP meetings even more than you do, so threatening them with another one can be effective.

Remember:

In the end, parents actually hold a lot of power in the IFSP and IEP processes. These plans are the federal government's attempt to force your school district to actually pay attention to your children's needs and puts parents in charge of deciding whether those needs are met. Lazy districts will take a "one size fits all" approach. Malevolent districts try to get their way by hustling, pressuring, and confusing parents about what choices are available and what their rights are. Bigoted districts will try to scare parents about the evils of sign language and Deaf culture. If you know that the process is *yours* and you know your rights, they will have a much harder time getting away with it. And if you have a good district, God bless you.

IFSPs in Yet More Excruciating Detail

Since most parents reading this book will be first dealing with an IFSP, here's a little more on the whole shebang.

IFSP Timeline

IDEA sets a very specific schedule for getting children an IFSP and then keeping it up to date.

- **Within two business days** of a diagnosis of "hearing loss," or another qualified disability, doctors, audiologists, or other professionals need to refer children to the state's Early Intervention program. Parents are free to self-refer as well, usually via the state's Early Intervention website.
- Districts then need to hold an *initial* or *intake* IFSP meeting, give all the needed assessments and tests, and write an IFSP with you **within forty-five days** of the referral date.
- Once an IFSP has been written, the district then needs to start services **as soon as possible**.
- IFSPs must be reviewed and updated **every six months** in an IFSP meeting. So if you sign your first IFSP on January 1, then you must have another scheduled *before* July 1.
- School districts must respond to IFSP requests made in writing **within ten business days** of getting the request.

- Parents can call additional IFSP meetings **whenever they need to**, if they feel services aren't being delivered or more / different services are needed.

- Your child must have a transition meeting to move from IFSP to IEP **between thirty and thirty-three months** (2 ½ to 2 ¾ years old) so they have an IEP ready to go at age three.

Speed is especially important given how slow identifying a deaf child can be, and how important early access to language is for them, so don't hesitate to hold your district to this schedule and call additional meetings if you need to. Always make your requests and document your issues via email so there's a record of them with a time and date attached.

First Contact: Intake Meetings

The *intake* or *initial* IFSP meeting is mostly for determining what assessments they should give your child that they haven't already, and for the school district to start pressuring you to use their cheapest in-house services. You'll meet with your district's team, which will consist of a service coordinator and at least one assessor, who's probably a teacher of the deaf (ToD) or a speech-language pathologist (SLP). You'll be asked to fill out one trillion consent forms, receive a bunch of more or less helpful pamphlets describing your rights, and answer questions to create a basic history about your kid's birth and health, your life at home, and your concerns about your child's development.

Remember that you only need to answer the questions you want to answer, and if they don't ask you something important, ask that they write it down as part of the IFSP. If you've made decisions about how you want to support your child already (for instance, with ASL), express them now and make sure they're actually recorded in the intake form.

Besides this interview, the district will also make a list of formal language and other developmental tests to give to your baby. Together, these two sets of assessments—your story and formal testing from professionals—will determine your child's goals and services in their first IFSP.

Be warned: some districts will play games with your child's disability definition under IDEA: kids with higher levels of residual hearing may get "hearing impaired" as their primary disability, but not "deaf"—this can be a problem, because without the *label* deaf, the district can try to withhold certain services or placements that your child needs. This is inappropriate, and actually against federal law, but fighting it after the fact sucks ass. Get "deaf" there.

This is also important if your child has multiple disabilities: if "deaf" isn't listed as the primary disability, districts can withhold related services that make school difficult or impossible. So even if your child has a disability in another area, think carefully how that will impact their *learning experience*. For some children, their other disability will take precedence, but for many, it's their deafness that will be the biggest obstacle.[20]

Remember that people you're meeting with might not have *much or any* experience with deaf children. Oscar's first service coordinator was a new hire from another district. She had plenty of special education experience and knew nothing about childhood deafness. On our way out of our first meeting, she asked *us* for the name of our local deaf services agency. SLPs and other assessors are sometimes the same—the average district sees very few deaf kids per year, and the vast majority of a pediatric SLP's patients are kids with typical hearing but other speech or language disorders. Ask how many deaf kids they have on their caseload and how many they serve annually.

In some ways, we were lucky to have a relatively blank slate to work with. Deaf education programs still graduate hundreds of oralist true believers each year, and professionals who have been working in the field can hold some shockingly outdated views of what deaf children need and are capable of, regardless of their experience. You need to be on the lookout for folks who might discourage ASL or other research-supported interventions for your kids, or who try to foist unproven (or disproven) methods like AVT or SEE sign.

What the IFSP team is required to tell you, but almost certainly won't emphasize, is *that you can bring your own people to an intake meeting*. Even if you think you're too far away from the deaf school, or if your kid has only mild

---

[20] Of course, districts love to play disabilities off against one another. "Oh, you requested an interpreter for your child's deafness. That means you don't get a classroom aide for their motor disability." No, fuckface, it means you get *both*.

or moderate levels of deafness, it's a good idea to contact them, or your local deaf services agency, and see if you can have an experienced Deaf educational advocate at the meeting. Unlike your local district people, deaf-ed advocates work with dozens of deaf kids and families on an annual basis and have a lot of experience, besides often being Deaf themselves and having firsthand knowledge to share. (Don't worry about communication, by the way: the district is required by law to supply an ASL interpreter if the meeting includes a Deaf attendee.) This "invite anyone" rule applies to other folks who'll be helpful: grandparents, Deaf relatives, any professionals you already know and trust. Don't be shy about bringing them along.

Meet the White Women

There's nothing wrong with white women—*I married one*—but special education in the United States is overwhelmingly staffed and administered by them, and as a profession, it has not distinguished itself in supporting families of color. Having a group of educators who know nothing about you or your family descend on your home and quiz you about how you're planning to raise your own child can be a problem, and you have the legal right to culturally competent support from your district, including materials in your home language. If you have concerns, get in touch with your local deaf services agency, and see if there's a local chapter of Black Deaf Advocates, Council De Manos, Asian Signers, and so on—they may have support, advice, and people for you.

Second Contact: Writing the IFSP

The Early Intervention team should try to set the first IFSP meeting as soon as possible after your intake meeting. They have forty-five days from the intake meeting to get the IFSP written, so they'll try to get any additional assessments needed done fast and then get you back for this.

This meeting is where you actually agree with the LEA on the services your child and your family will receive from the district. Just like at intake, you have the right to have anyone there who can comment on your child's needs and well-being. The more of your people in the room, or in the Zoom, the better. If you weren't able to have a Deaf educational advocate at the intake, bring them now if you can—district representatives who are used to going unchallenged will have a lot harder time lying, exaggerating, or omitting information when faced with someone who knows the score.

This meeting is also the moment to start picking your people and weeding out the folks you don't trust. Watch how they talk to you and how they talk about your child. Look out for anyone who's contradicting or undermining your decisions. Professionals who have concerns should be expressing them with you before the meeting to give you time to understand and respond to their concerns. Anyone who's an obstacle in the meeting, or who is condescending toward you or your kid, or sets low expectations for them, shouldn't be invited back—if you can't switch to a new provider, at least have them send a written report and not come to the meeting itself. See the section *Dealing with Bad Professionals* for more info. **Although you might feel very unsure about yourself, you are in charge.**

Third Contact and So on . . . IFSP's Until Age Three

Once the IFSP has been written, you'll start having them at six-month intervals. In each meeting, you and your team should be discussing the progress your child has made on their goals, the effectiveness of the various services you got, and adding (or subtracting) anything from the plans that you need.

The IEP Transition Meeting

The move from IFSP to IEP is a big fat hairy deal. This is the time when school placement decisions start getting made, so the district will really put the screws on you to mainstream your kid—see the section *Placement, FAPE, and the Problem with LRE* for more details. This is also the moment when everything shifts to a "deficit model"; you'll have to start phrasing assessments a lot more carefully in order to get what your child needs.

It may also involve a change of staff, from the Early Intervention people to the district's special education or deaf education unit, so you could be dealing with a whole new set of administrators and professionals—often this is when what's been a friendly relationship with a district turns adversarial.

For my son, it included all sorts of new testing with unfamiliar SLPs and educational psychologists.

This is why telling the story of where you want your child to go and why asking for all the services your child needs in the IFSP is critical. If you've had a good time of it so far, those friendly faces from Early Intervention may suddenly disappear, and if a district doesn't want to support your child with services like an interpreter, or if they're opposed to sending your kid to the deaf school or other appropriate program, they will use the history of your IFSP against you.

Parents also need to be ready for the shift away from family-based services:

The IEP transition is often where parents stumble and struggle. Whatever services they were getting under the IFSP are now no longer available to the family. This is a harsh realization for parents to come to terms with while navigating a whole new system within the IEP realm. It is really important to identify who your village members are to support you when the transition occurs.

Susan Gonzalez, Deaf educational advocate

Assessments, Services, and Goals for IFSPs and IEPs

Assessments

These can come in different forms, but they are either written observations by you, your kid's therapists, teachers, or caregivers, or school grades, or other formal tests of your child's development. Taken altogether, the assessments will then be used to determine what goals you set for your child.

Written observations will be a general description of your child and their behavior, plus notes from your kids' medical record and audiology report, and a brief description of your child's history and family situation—parents and siblings, caregivers, and what their home environment is like. For tests, there is a wide range of formal assessments that could be used, depending on the particulars of your child and what the assessors are accustomed to doing. In particular, testers need to be trained in administering and interpreting tests for deaf children and need to give tests that are *normed* for deaf kids—where some baseline expectations for deaf children have been established. For instance, deaf kids' spatial reasoning skills are generally more advanced than hearing kids their age, so any test that measures these skills needs to take that into account. Language First maintains an ongoing list of these assessments on their website.

While these kinds of assessments can seem very neutral and scientific, in truth they're only approximations and are influenced by the assessor's own biases and background. This is why parents are encouraged to add their own observations to the IFSP/IEP and to recruit their own professionals to do assessments if they feel like they need outside expertise. Districts must accept assessments from qualified professionals, and they need to be able to tell you what "qualified" means—typically anyone licensed to work in your state.

Services

The "Individual" in IFSP means that you can ask for essentially any service for your child or your family that will improve their long-term academic, social-emotional, and quality of life outcomes. When your child moves to IEPs, you have to focus more narrowly on them and their *academic* issues, but this still includes things like their social experiences and psychological well-being at school.

This also means you don't have to just take what's offered by your district: the district can pay for outside resources, classes, and therapies if they don't offer them in-house. The district may not be *eager* to pay for these outside services, or even know they exist, so it's important to ask around. Check your deaf services agency, outreach at your local deaf school (even if it's on the other side of the state), other parents of deaf kids in your area, any Deaf adults you know, outside professionals you trust, and hit up Google, too.

Remember that the "Family" part means that it's not just services for your child—you, your spouse, or partner, and your other children can all get services through the IFSP if it helps you support your deaf baby.

Here's a *very* partial list of services that you can advocate for in an IFSP:

- Language and other assessments from district professionals (ToDs, SLPs, etc.)

- Language and other assessments from qualified outside professionals that *you* choose
- Placement in specialized DHH preschools and programs in your school district
- Placement in specialized DHH preschools and programs *outside of your district or state*
- In-home visits from teachers of the deaf (ToDs)
- In-home visits from Deaf mentors or Deaf coaches
- Educational ASL interpreters for mainstream settings, from daycare onwards
- ASL classes or educational subsidies for you, your family, and your child
- Speech-language pathology services and therapy for English
- Speech-language pathology services and therapy for ASL
- Speech-language pathology services and therapy for your home language
- Literacy and reading support services
- Physical therapy (PT) services
- Occupational therapy (OT) services
- Psychiatric services
- Orientation and mobility services for DeafBlind or low-vision kids
- ProTactile or Tactile ASL language instruction for DeafBlind or low-vision kids
- Intervenor services for deafblind kids in mainstream or deaf-ed settings, from daycare onward
- Braille literacy services for DeafBlind or low-vision kids
- Music, art, dance, or sports classes for audio, visual, occupational, or physical rehabilitation
- Access to specialized parenting classes or support groups for you or your family

- Transportation subsidies to get your kid to school or services, including vouchers for gas money and door-to-door busing / taxi services
- Childcare subsidies to get respite care or time to take classes / receive services
- Subsidies for DHH family camps or other remote events to receive more training and support

Most of these services are available for IEPs, too. IEP services can only go to your child, **but that includes anything that impacts your child's academic experience and ability to learn at school**. Your kid's social-emotional development, their physical and psychiatric well-being, as well as any academic needs, are all fair game for an IEP-related service.

Now it's true that the district may not have quality services to offer, and your LEA may not give you everything you ask for anyway. Specific rules and guidelines vary state to state and region to region. However, your district is *guaranteed* not to give you services that you don't ask for.

Case in point: during Covid lockdown, our son was stuck in the house with his hearing family, and because he was separated from most of the fluent signers in his life, his ASL hit a plateau. When school restarted, we went to our next meeting and asked the LEA for speech-language pathology services to help him work on his expressive ASL.

The LEA: "We don't do speech-language pathology for ASL."

My wife: "That's funny, because he's got a documented language delay in the language of instruction at a state school that you guys agreed to send him to. If the language delay were in English, you wouldn't hesitate for a second."

In the end, the LEA found a little money in the budget for an ASL SLP after all. I *love* my wife.

What gets written into the first IFSP is going to have a powerful effect on your child's education going forward, so I strongly recommend bringing your checklist of services and any specific things you want written into the doc.

At a minimum, you should advocate for the following in your IFSP:

- Weekly sessions and regular assessments in all your chosen languages by SLPs who know those languages and are experienced in pediatric deafness

- Weekly visits with a qualified ToD to assess and support language acquisition in English, ASL, or whatever languages you're focusing on
- Deaf mentoring or coaching for the family if available
- ASL classes or education for your family (in-person or remote—don't let them tell you nobody does this in your district)
- Placement in a specialized DHH day program / preschool if you have one nearby—even if it's across state lines
- Transit services or reimbursement for any commute you need to do with your kid

I recommend not signing the IFSP during the meeting itself. Take the document home with you at the end of the session to read over in a lower-pressure environment and consult your favorite pros if you have questions. Send any edits or additions back to the entire team via email and get it looking like you want. Once you're satisfied, then sign and return so you can start services.

Remote Services and Online Learning

Before 2019, you were often out of luck if there wasn't a professional in your area who could offer a given therapy / class. While there were a few remote programs, most therapists and educators only worked face-to-face and tended to cluster around deaf schools or cities with large populations. If you lived out on the farm and needed support, there might be no options but relocating your family, waiting for rare visits from providers, or making long or even overnight commutes.

Then Covid showed up. Suddenly, *everyone* had to figure out how to do as much as possible online. It was rough for a while—Oscar's providers saw him perform a lot of pants-free gymnastics in the early days of lockdown—but necessity is the mother of invention. These days, many professionals have solid remote-work methods and see part or all of their clients via Zoom or similar. This can be a lifeline for families for many reasons, and it makes rural living a lot more doable.

Remote services aren't just for folks out in the country, though. Even if you live in town, they can be the only way to access certain things your district just doesn't have, especially around ASL-based therapies, where many districts offer diddly-squat. If your kid is medically fragile, doing as much as possible online can help protect them from Covid or other health hazards they might encounter out in the world. And remote services are also helpful when you need to find that purple squirrel—a rare pro with exactly the right mix of skills, like a Deaf ASL instructor who also knows Cantonese for grandma.

Remote is not a cure-all; besides districts just refusing services out of policy, cost, or bigotry, there are services that can't be done reliably online, and some kids just don't work well on the computer. My own son enjoys English speech therapy remotely—and even though we've been back in school for years now, he still does it by Zoom out of convenience. But for ASL, he really needs support face-to-face. And generally, the younger your child is, the more in-person contact is needed for services to be effective. This means that when the professional is on the far end of the camera, it falls to parents to be more actively involved in order to make it work—no goofing off on your phone while your kid is in session.

Remote services also require a newish computer and a solid internet connection. These are things you can ask the district to help with as part of your IFSP / IEP. You might also find a sufficiently high-speed hookup at your local library or even at a district school—if a remote service is in your IFSP or IEP, your district will need to find you a sufficiently fast connection if you don't have it at home.

If you want to include remote services in your IFSP/ IEP, it's not typically a problem if the professional works for your district—just talk with them about how they operate, and you can make a plan. If the remote service is coming from an out-of-district provider, you'll often be challenged to justify outside help versus taking what the district has to offer. Which brings us to . . .

Third Party Assessment and Services

IDEA guarantees that you can get a second opinion for any assessments the district has already done, or assessments for things the district doesn't know how to do. And because you need to get testing done before you can get a service provided, if there's any gap in the district's services, assessment is the first step to getting that service from a third party. Most qualified assessors are also service providers, so testing can become a little bit of a dating game between your district and these outside professionals.

Our district offered SLP services in English, but we were raising Oscar bilingual and wanted the district to test his ASL development, too. When we went to the district's speech-language pathologist, she suggested, and I shit you not, that the Deaf secretary at the local day program give the assessment. Instead, we began a multi-month search for a qualified ASL-fluent speech-language pathologist. It turns out that there were actually two in the Bay Area: one was an hour away by car, and the other was *two* hours away. But since nobody in our district had any training in ASL-based language development, in the end they agreed to pay for one of them to drive up and do the testing.

Once an assessment has identified an area where your child has needs, you then need to bring the test back to an IFSP or IEP meeting, hopefully along with the assessor or other professional you want to work with. The LEA then needs to make a decision on whether the district will pay this person or not. If the district determines that the service is necessary, and that they don't have any way of providing the same service in-house, and that they have the money to pay for it, then you might get your third party. This is exactly what happened in our case: the assessing SLP attended the meeting, testified that our guy needed extra ASL support, and was eventually added as a third-party provider.

Writing IFSP and IEP Goals

Your kid's goals for an IFSP or IEP can be language-based, cognitive, academic, social-emotional, physical, or occupational—any category where your kid may need support. They should also be written in a particular way:

Goals must be *specific and measurable*—they say explicitly what has to happen, have a time period when it must happen, plus a number, percentage, or proportion of times it must happen. If it's a language goal, they should always refer to a *specific* language. And goals must always say *who* is doing the measuring: which teacher, therapist, or parent is keeping track.

A good goal will look something like this:

Baby X will correctly label emotions for self and others<—***specific goal*** in ASL<—***specific language*** 80% of the time when asked<—***measurable number*** over a period of two weeks<—***time period*** as confirmed by SLP observation<—***person doing the measuring.***

or

Baby X will spontaneously use an English vocabulary of between 15-20 words over the course of a month as documented by preschool staff.

Baby X will demonstrate proficient use of a sippy cup in 3 out of 4 trials over the course of 8 weeks as documented by the occupational therapist.

Baby X will maintain an upright sitting position in at least 3 separate sessions for at least 10 seconds, as recorded by the physical therapy team.

If your team is writing goals that don't include *how often, how much,* and *who,* bring that up in the meeting and get it corrected in the plan. Professionals should be keeping records of their activities with your kid. Properly written goals can be checked against those records to hold the district accountable—if the services are being provided but the goals aren't being met, you can demand more or different services. And as always, for deaf children, focus on functional language goals.

504 Plans: If You Really Loved Me, You Wouldn't Hurt Me

504 plans come from Section 504 of *The Rehabilitation Act of 1973*. This was the first federal law that mandated public education for children with disabilities. At the time, it was revolutionary,[21] and it anchors many basic rights for deaf children, but 504 plans themselves have been superseded by the much more helpful and comprehensive plans established in IDEA. 504s are particularly pushed on children transitioning out of an IFSP, as an alternative to an IEP, but don't fall for it—compared with IEPs, they suck:

---

[21] The film *Crip Camp* gives a riveting account of the 504 sit-ins. It's absolutely required watching.

- 504s only cover your local public school district—no special school placements

- Third-party assessments aren't available unless the family pays for them, although testing by in-school or in-district folks like SLPs or PTs might be included

- There may be no mandated structure or schedules for a 504 in your state—depending on state law, plans might not even need to be written down

- The appeals process for a 504 gives you fewer options between "complaining to the school" and "filing an actual goddamn lawsuit under federal civil rights law"

- Instead of having a list of specific disabilities, 504s cover *any* disability that interferes with a child's ability to learn in a general education environment

Given these differences, and the fact that "deafness," "deafblindness," and "hearing impairment" are all specifically listed as qualifying disabilities under IDEA for IFSPs and IEPs, there is almost no reason for you to choose a 504 for your child.

However, school district officials *love* 504s because they're much less work, with less oversight, and fewer expensive obligations. Once your kid is on a 504, you're relying entirely on your local school's competence and benevolence to make sure they get appropriate accommodations. The process of filing complaints for 504s is basically, "if you can't settle it inside the school's complaint system, go to your local Office of Civil Rights." On the one hand, the district has less power to tie you up in procedural hearings, as in an IFSP or IEP, but on the other, you've basically got to be willing to go to the mat and sue their ass for violations. In short, if your LEA tries to sell you on a 504, call them a neckless dweeb and demand your IEP.

The only area where a 504 outshines an IEP is in its definition of disability: if your kid somehow doesn't meet the criteria under IDEA's thirteen categories of disability (as interpreted by your state), you can still likely get a 504 plan. If that's the case, you can appeal their decision (educational advocate time!), but you may need to settle for a 504 in the meantime in order to get in-class accommodations like special seating, FM systems, or ASL interpreters.

Some kids get good and necessary services from 504s, but those are typically in cases where a child doesn't need placement in a deaf program, and teachers don't need a lot of specialized knowledge, and you have a trusting relationship with your teachers and district. For deaf kids, this ain't the norm.

Dealing with Bad Professionals

Therapists, doctors, and educators work for you.[22] This is true whether they're an SLP, ToD, PT, OT, ENT, AuD, pediatrician, interpreter, or whatever, and it's true whether they come to you through your school district, early intervention, your insurance company, or if you pay their bill out of pocket. Parents often feel stuck with a bad service provider, especially if they're assigned by the district, but if they are misbehaving or not giving your child what they need, you have the legal right to tell them to shape up. If they don't, firing a shitty pro is the sweetest feeling in the world.

There's a sliding scale for handling rogue providers, depending on how badly they are acting, what your overall tolerance is for their shenanigans, and whether you can get the same services someplace else. Nobody gets into this business if they don't care about kids, but good intentions don't mean they aren't carrying harmful assumptions about deaf children and language acquisition. Bad professionals can use "saving the poor deaf babies" as an excuse for atrocious behavior that can do lasting damage to your kid.

Correcting the Profesh

On the gentler end of things, you might only need to ask a professional to behave professionally. People are going to judge you—that's the reality of having kids—but we're asking for *silent* judgment. A pediatrician who makes an offhand remark about your child "not needing sign language" may just

---

[22] Actually, they work for *your child*, but you're the one calling the shots right now.

need to be reminded of his bedside manner: "Please don't discuss our family's language choices during the visit—we work with language development specialists to make our decisions."

Particularly if yours is the first deaf kid they have ever seen, a kind but direct correction can bring someone around who's just parroting bad advice and secondhand bias. Remember that whatever degree they might hold, you're often arriving at appointments with more education and real-world perspective than they are:

> Pediatric certification for audiology is rigorous. Unfortunately, not a single aspect of certification addresses signed languages, the Deaf community, or Deaf Education. This is why so many pediatric audiologists, even in large facilities like Children's Hospitals, still have no understanding of the educational system their patients will interface with, and no understanding of how language development (and lack thereof) can impact educational outcomes for Deaf children.
>
>   Mallorie Evans, Audiologist and Professor of Deaf Education

It pays to pick your moment for a correction; unless you see something that needs immediate attention, wait until the end of the appointment itself, or ask for a few minutes before the next session to discuss your concern. Let them know that the comment or behavior was not appropriate, explain why, and ask that they not do it again. This gives the provider a chance to focus on what you're saying and models for them the kind of respectful interaction you expect in return.

You can also put your request into an email afterward, which can give you time to choose your words and organize your thoughts. Even if you've already spoken to the pro, it's important to also send a polite follow-up email, repeating what you said, why you said it, and thanking the provider in advance. These emails are time-stamped records of your interactions, and **written records of any kind are critical if you need to file an administrative or legal complaint later.** Even if you feel like you missed your moment and didn't say something when you should have, you should still write down any misbehavior, along with the date, and keep it handy for later.

Law and Order: SLP

The "calm correction" approach is great when it works, especially if you're only visiting once a year for shots and a checkup. But if you're seeing a provider more often, and they're not taking the hint, you may need to escalate.

Oscar's very first speech-language pathologist seemed great. "June" was our school district's pick for IFSP services in spoken English. She'd been with early intervention for years, and she was a high-energy, rainbow overalls kind of therapist. We loved the enthusiasm, and she quickly connected with baby Oscar, but there were problems from the beginning. In her first assessment, she wrote that we were using total communication with Oscar—this wasn't correct, and we sent back the first draft. She left it in the second draft. We asked her to correct it again.

"Oh I'm sorry, I've just never heard of bilingual deaf education."

It soon became clear that this was bullshit. June did not like ASL, held a low opinion of Deaf adults, and never missed an opportunity to tell us about their tragic and deprived lives. This was shocking to my wife and me, because she treated plenty of deaf kids and had a number of Deaf colleagues. (She also advised my wife to quit her job to help care for Oscar, which was bizarre because it was her job that paid the bills and carried the insurance.) But because June seemed to make progress with Oscar, and because we had no idea what our rights really were, we let her weirdness go.

During the next regular IFSP meeting, we sat down with June, the LEA, and the rest of Oscar's treatment team, and presented what we thought was a solid plan: Oscar would spend thirty hours a week with a Deaf nanny to get fluent ASL exposure. He'd spend the rest of his time at home with us, and we would give him English exposure, take him to weekly SLP and ToD sessions, and work on our ASL together. Both June and Oscar's ToD agreed that he was progressing in all his expected milestones for language acquisition, for both English and ASL, and that there were no concerns with the plan.

It was very fast and easy until it was over. We'd finished approving goals and services, signed the IFSP, and had formally ended the session. Then, just before we got up to leave, June piped up:

"I'm just worried about this Deaf babysitter of yours. 30 hours a week in *silence*? Why don't you just get a hearing interpreting student? They can talk *and* sign; they don't even really have to be fluent in ASL."

For which she got a bunch of nodding heads, and *oh yeah, I was worried about that*'s from the LEA and assembled team.

In hindsight, I can tell you exactly what was wrong with a move like this:

- Slipping her opinion in *after* the meeting ended so we couldn't object or discuss it
- Abusing her authority in front of our clueless LEA and the rest of the IFSP team
- Undercutting our stated goals as parents
- Trying to deprive our son of fluent language models
- Pretending ASL isn't a language because it isn't spoken
- Being a thunderous farting asshole of a human being

At the time, though, it felt like we'd stepped in a bear trap.

So after the IFSP, my wife and I contacted our local deaf services agency and spoke with their educational advocate. With her help and advice, we decided that there would be no more ambushes. June could continue to work with Oscar, but we would ask her to submit written reports to us ahead of time and never attend another IFSP meeting. Meanwhile, my wife called every speech-language pathologist in the Bay Area, looking for someone willing to work with a bilingual family.

I took Oscar to a few more appointments, and June kept on working with him, and she brought the same Ms. Rachel enthusiasm to our sessions as before. Then it was my wife's turn. This was a few weeks before the next IFSP meeting, so she brought up the topic of sending written recommendations instead of attending. That was when June made her feelings known: about how *betrayed* she felt and how she meant no *disrespect*—other families *loved* her. I was the easy one to work with, why was my wife so *hard* (as if we hadn't made the decision together)? Wasn't supporting Oscar *the most important thing*?

My wife replied that, frankly, her behavior was inappropriate and bigoted, which is why we were asking for a little distance. So June stormed out. She stormed back in. She cried. She shouted. She fired *us*.

The end result was a formal complaint to June's employer, an abject apology from her supervisor (with a big helping of "please don't sue us" on the side), and an appointment with a new speech-language pathologist paid for by our insurance. This new SLP didn't sign or use ASL in any way, but she was more than happy to work with Oscar on his receptive and expressive English, and she did not give two shits about what he did with the rest of his time.

And that is how we fired our first professional.

Ready . . . Aim . . .

Because they work for your child, you can always just tell a pro to take a hike if you think your kid would be better off without them. But to successfully fire a therapist or educator and *continue to get those services paid for by the district*, you first need to document the provider acting out. Every time you see *the behavior,* write it down, along with the date and your polite-but-firm objection. You need all three parts there so that nobody can play the idiot; there's a record that you expressed your wishes and that the professional ignored them.

I'd recommend giving a bad pro *one* warning. The first time you catch something shady happening, make your complaint and put it in an email to the professional. The second time, make your complaint to the provider, and cc the email to their boss and the district LEA. The "fool me once" policy is important because some of the worst offenders are frog boilers. They will constantly look for ways to undermine you, slowly turning up the heat; setting expectations early is a lot easier than climbing out of a pot of hot frog soup. In retrospect, we could have saved ourselves trouble if we'd given June some pushback early on.

However, if you catch a professional crossing any of the red lines below, that's an automatic out; document it and call an IFSP / IEP meeting right away; do not wait for the next regular meeting and do not return for another appointment.

Call for Backup

When you first smell a rotten pro, it's time to take stock of the entire educational pantry, your insurance coverage, and your personal budget. Start talking with other parents and reach out to organizations like the American Society for Deaf Children, the American Board of DHH Specialists, or Language First, which keeps lists of "pro-ASL" professionals for each state on their website. Depending on where you live and what the service is, there may be other, better folks working for your school district or in adjacent districts, or regional programs that your family qualifies for—sometimes the school district isn't the only game in town.

There may also be private practitioners that you can turn to, locally or remotely. Deaf-savvy providers keep track of one another, so reach out even if you think they aren't available—they may have a colleague who is. Check with your insurance, too. We were very surprised when our policy agreed to pay for Oscar's SLP services, and very happy with the office they referred us to.

When you find someone that fits your kid's needs, ask if they have already done work for your school district. There is a vetting process for outside providers who get paid through IFSP / IEP plans. If this professional has already gotten approved in the past, getting your child's services moved to them will be less of a fight.

Call the Meeting

Once you know how you want things to go—whether you need another practitioner from inside the district, or if you need the district to pay an outsider, or if you or your insurance are footing the bill—call an IFSP / IEP meeting by sending an email requesting one to your district LEA. Describe the misbehavior you encountered and state that you are looking for a resolution to the issue. Ask that the professional not attend, but bring along any allies you have, like a Deaf educational advocate, your child's other caregivers, or other folks. Be aware that friendly professionals, even if they agree with you, aren't always that helpful in these situations. They need to protect their relationship with the district and generally show more respect and deference to colleagues than is useful when what you're planning is a murder.

At the meeting, present your evidence—each incident along with your response—in writing to the LEA, and ask to change providers. You will probably get pushback: your current provider is the cheapest and easiest option for them, so they may not want to transfer your kid to another in-district provider, let alone go through the headache of sending your kid to a neighboring district. LEAs are generally loath to pay for third parties if they can help it. Remember, though, that they are required by law to provide services listed in the IEP one way or another. Your goal is to show them a piece of paper with a bunch of incriminating evidence on it and let them run the costs in their head: price and hassle of a different provider versus price and hassle of a lawsuit.[23]

Results, Mixed, and Otherwise

IDEA lets you pick assessors and demand appropriate services, but it doesn't guarantee you get the providers you ask for. You need to be prepared to compromise: if there's another professional in the district, or one that's already working with your child that can do the thing, the LEA will almost certainly move those goals over to them even if they're not your first choice. But if nobody else in the district can provide the service, you may hit the jackpot. Have your list of pros ready; you're probably the only one who's done any research, so if you hand them a couple of reasonable options, that might carry the day. But your LEA may decide to call your bluff and let the shit professional off with a warning, despite the evidence. In that case, here are your options:

Continue to see the pro, and hope the meeting was sufficient to keep them in line. However bland the LEA seemed at the meeting, I guarantee that the conversation they had with the provider beforehand was spicy. If they step out of line again, write it down and call another meeting, and bring an educational advocate or lawyer this time. Rinse and repeat. If the district doesn't change your provider after a second meeting, you're probably on your way to a formal civil rights complaint or lawsuit.

---

[23]Remember that the Supreme Court has now ruled in *Luna Perez vs. Sturgis Public Schools* that districts are liable for monetary damages for harm they do to deaf children, even if they settle educational issues under IDEA.

Stop seeing the pro and get private or other services not managed by your district. If you've got the money, or a solid insurance policy, or there's another regional service you can access, it's a nice choice to have.

Stop seeing the pro and go without. It's not a great option, but you might decide that it's worth the trade-off. Continuing to see a persistently abusive professional can do enormous harm to your child (and to you). Sometimes nothing is the best thing, at least for the time being.

Escalate inside the system and register a formal complaint. Keep in mind that formal complaints under IDEA are handled differently by different districts, but they are not a fast, fun, or cheap process. You will certainly need an educational advocate or lawyer to be successful at this level. School districts can drag their feet for *years* on complaints, and your child needs support *now*. If you arrive at this stage, you should seriously look at ditching the district if you can—either moving or enrolling elsewhere. It's not fair, but if these services are critical to your child's well-being, you don't have time to fuck around.

In our case, we've pretty much done one of everything *except* move. We've had goals transferred to another in-district team member, we've had the district pay for an outside provider, we've made a formal complaint, and we've had to go back to a professional who was warned, hoping that the shit-fit we threw was enough to keep them in line.

Red Flags

Often the first sign of trouble from a provider is a comment that reveals ignorance or bias.

- "You're only hard of hearing—you don't need to be with those *deaf* kids over there."
- "She should be in a normal class." (when *normal = mainstream*)
- "He needs to practice being around hearing kids because it's a hearing world."
- "Everyone loves him, he has so many friends." (or other forms of empty-ass flattery)

"We will see if she needs sign language."

"He can hear me just fine, he's just not paying attention."

"Learn ASL? No, we don't teach second languages here."

"If you're not going to make them wear their HAs / CIs, that's like child abuse."

"Oh she speaks so well, you don't even know she's deaf."

"If she learns ASL, no one else will know it." (total bullshit, by the way—ASL ranks third behind Spanish and French in most-studied languages in US higher education.)

Red Lines

If the phrases above signal trouble, any of the actions below merit an immediate meeting with the LEA.

Violating the terms of the IFSP / IEP. If the plan says X, but then they drop X or switch to Y without consulting you. This covers methods: if they say they are going to use ASL and then they talk; if you ask them not cover their mouth for speech, and then they cover it, and so on. It applies to changes to timing or frequency: if a professional is missing multiple appointments, or regularly cuts sessions short, or reduces the number of weekly meetings without informing you. It also applies to goals: particularly if your child isn't going to meet a goal outlined in their plan, or needs to modify a goal or service for any reason, you should know about it long in advance of the next IFSP / IEP meeting, and have already discussed and approved it with the pro ahead of time, not when you're sitting down with the district.

Undermining your parental rights. This isn't just a difference of opinion, it's when the professional uses their leverage to interfere with or undo decisions you've already made. Last-minute meetings or changes to a plan, misrepresenting your words or the advice of other professionals, leaving critical information out of reports, using emotionally manipulative language to your face or in written communications, going behind your back to other members of your child's treatment team, and so on. IDEA gives you clear rights as a parent, and there are a million underhanded ways they can be taken from you.

> My district used to cancel meetings they felt would be confrontational, and make parents miss work for nothing, until they couldn't miss any more work. Then we'd hold the meeting without the parents.
>
> Anonymous mainstream ToD

Disparaging deaf people. It doesn't matter if your kid is seeing a hardcore no-signing AVT speech-language pathologist—*hearing professionals do not speak badly of deaf people and their choices*, and they do not speak badly of Deaf culture or ASL in front of you or your child. If they disagree with a particular practice or approach, they can say things like, "I don't think that's effective," and leave it there. Remember, whatever they say about another deaf person, they are potentially saying about *your baby*.

Deaf professionals get more leeway with this, but even then, the focus should be on your kid and their needs, and what programs or practices they think would help most.

Harming your child in any way. Therapy should never be punitive or painful, and if you catch a therapist doing anything questionable, yank your kid out of there and report the behavior to the provider's manager and to the district LEA.

"Harm" definitely means hitting or yelling, but also includes manipulative language like, "if you were a *good* boy, you would say the word," or trying to force unwilling babies and toddlers to do drills or perform behaviors they are too exhausted or frustrated to do, or forcing them to keep devices on when they don't want to, or using any tactic that relies on shame, fear, or pain. Not only is this abusive, it just isn't an effective teaching tool compared with gentle, play-based methods.

Reporting abuse to the LEA and the provider's supervisor in writing is key. Send an email that explicitly says, "I saw your provider hurting my child," and detail the inappropriate behavior you saw or know about and demand that they take legal action. These folks are almost certainly *mandatory reporters*, meaning they must, by law, start an investigation with the proper authorities.

If you don't get an immediate answer, go up the chain again and talk to the boss's boss, and keep going. Abuse happens, but you don't have to tolerate it.

Schools, Preschools, Daycares, and Sitters

Because of their small number and varied quality, picking the right school or program for your baby is going to shape their future more than any other decision you make. It's going to shape your life, too: you may find yourself hauling ass halfway across the state on a daily basis, changing jobs, and otherwise scrambling your plans to get your child what they need. What a quality education gives your kid, though, is worth it, because education for deaf children is the gateway to independence, opportunity, friendship, and growth for deaf adults.

Three Is the Magic Number

When thinking about different kinds of care and school situations for deaf children, from infancy onward, it's helpful to divide their needs into three areas:

Body (basic care): Your child needs to be kept safe and healthy at all times. Diapers changed, meals provided, boo-boos kissed, wolves chased away. This is the bedrock minimum, and unfortunately, even this can be a struggle for many families in our shitty system.

Mind (language exposure): Accessible language exposure is the first essential education your baby is going to need, so if you are using ASL with your child, getting them into an environment with fluent signers is important. This isn't sitting in a chair getting drilled by a teacher or therapist; it's playing with friends and teachers, making messes and cleaning them up, eating, drinking, and pooping, and observing other people using language. As your child gets older, the ABCs, counting, and other types of more classroom-y learning become important and are enabled by your kid's early access to language.

Spirit (socialization): Babies need baby friends and sweet-natured adults to practice being human with. Hearing friends are good, but as your child grows, having deaf peers and role models will be important to help them figure out how to interact with the world and have healthy relationships and self-worth. This is the most "woo" of the needs, but it's real and important to their long-term happiness. Yours, too; kids who don't develop strong social skills and self-esteem struggle to get shit done in their lives. It's a one-way ticket to living in your basement.

In a perfect world, you'll be able to meet all three needs in one place. A signing daycare, preschool, or kindergarten where you can drop off your child for as long as you need, where they have exposure to fluent ASL and deaf peers and teachers they can directly communicate with.

In reality, you might find yourself handing over your child to a hearing daycare or non-signing relative or sitter for most of their day, only to get ASL exposure for a fraction of the day at a parent and child class, and only see deaf peers on the weekends or playdates. As they get older, they may spend more time in a DHH classroom, but still be in a hearing afterschool or other situation. You'll likely need to hustle up a patchwork of different services to cover everything, and resolve this particular Rubik's cube a couple of times before your child even starts kindergarten.

Options for Infants and Toddlers

Baby care in the United States sucks, and for deaf babies, it's no different—the unspoken assumption is that a parent (aka a mother) is going to somehow magically be free to watch any kid under the age of two. That said, the situation improves as time goes on.

Your options are going to be essentially random, determined by what resources you have and can dig up in your area. My family solved the issue with money and luck by finding a Deaf nanny to take Oscar for most of the day, with me taking up the slack and eventually leaving my job to manage things. When my son turned three, he qualified for our local deaf school's Early Childhood Education program (ECE).

Bilingual Infant and Toddler Programs/Early Childhood Education

For our son, the early childhood center at the deaf school was the golden ticket. The ticket to language, the ticket to social skills and acceptance—everything.

John, hearing father

If you can find them, an ASL-based bilingual early childhood education program is going to be the best option. These are often run out of state deaf schools, but are sometimes found in other school districts or via EI. For infants, programs generally require parents to be in attendance, although grandparents or other caregivers are welcome, too. As your child gets older, drop-off programs become available, although not always full-day; here in California, the state deaf schools can only look after two-year-olds for twelve hours per week by law, which scales up to thirty hours per week for five-year-olds / kindergarteners, so finding additional care to plug that gap is a challenge.

Hearing Daycares and Preschools

Maybe the easiest care to find for your kid (although "easy" sometimes means long waiting lists or outrageous tuition fees) is a run-of-the-mill daycare operated by hearing staff. These programs can certainly care for your child's body, and there is definitely some learning and socialization that can happen, especially if your child has access to spoken language. But if your child needs ASL, they are a big blank spot. You will need to find another source of ASL exposure, and may want to limit the amount of time your child spends in that linguistic dead zone if you can.

If you need to place your kid in a hearing daycare, you can use your IFSP to get educational interpreters, itinerant ToDs, and Deaf mentors visiting with your child in school from the very beginning. Also, explore getting their hearing staff more training; there may be resources available from your local deaf services agency if the owner or program director is interested in leveling up their skills. Although nobody is going to become a language model, basic correct sign language for the staff will help with day-to-day care and inclusion for your child.

Hearing Sitters, Nannies, and Grannies

Same as above, really. A loving hearing caregiver can give your child a lot—but they can't give them sign language exposure. You can potentially have a nanny or relative bring your child to drop-in sessions at your local deaf school or service agency, though, or even take independent ASL classes (that *you* pay for). It's not a replacement for learning ASL yourself, but it will help your child develop their language and build your sitter's ability to communicate with your kid, and it can be a good part of the overall package.

Because, well, family, beware of stubborn z-holes who refuse to learn ASL or otherwise won't get with the program. See *Language Lessons for Late Learners* for more on them.

"Vanilla" Special Education Programs

Your district may have options for drop-off care via Early Intervention, but beware: districts sometimes take a one-size-fits-all approach and shunt deaf kids into special education environments alongside children with vastly different needs—I've seen programs that put sighted deaf children alongside hearing kids who are blind, and mixing neurotypical deaf children who sign with neurodivergent hearing kids who don't.

While maximizing inclusion is often a good strategy for kids with a wide array of disabilities, and deaf children can benefit from social peers of all kinds—hearing and deaf, disabled and not—deaf *education* is a highly specialized field. These programs might incorporate some kind of sign system like SEE, but for kids who need ASL exposure, these programs can be linguistic dead zones, too. Unfortunately, these are often the locations where the district hosts their SLPs, ToDs, and so on; but unless you're looking at a real bilingual program, these are more like hearing daycares and don't provide strong language exposure or good role models.

Oral DHH Daycares and Preschools

These are programs run along oral-education philosophies, typically Listening and Spoken Language. You can see my notes about oral programs below—I generally think that these are not the best options for many kids, and that you're exposing them to higher risks in terms of both language deprivation and social-emotional development. These schools can *look* very slick, though; they will focus on speech and hearing training and generally integrate speech-language pathology and other forms of therapy into the day. Expect them to frown on ASL and discourage its use at school (and possibly outside school too), and for the teachers and staff to be majority hearing.

Signing Daycares and Preschools

You'll occasionally find a licensed in-home daycare or nursery school run by a Deaf or CODA person, where they use ASL as the daily language. If you can locate something like this, it's a great choice to get your kid fluent exposure to ASL. These are typically small private businesses, relying on word-of-mouth, although the local deaf school or deaf services agency may know about them. They're rare, and they may not be the most polished, fru-fru option in your area. Nevertheless, kids don't mind shabby toys or the lack of in-house SLPs one bit, and as long as the environment is safe and loving, and they are truly using ASL most of the day, they can be a great choice and meet the care / language / socialization threebie effortlessly. Because they don't have the same restrictions as state-run programs, they are also useful for enrolling hearing siblings to get them ASL exposure, too!

In our area, an established preschool has set up a separate ASL program, staffed by Deaf teachers and volunteers, that coordinates with the deaf school's early childhood center to cover the workday. Kids are dropped at the deaf school's toddler program by parents, bussed to the preschool, and picked up in the evening again by parents.

Deaf and Signing Nannies, Sitters, and Grannies

For meeting the mind and soul bits of the equation, an ASL-fluent caregiver is amazing. If they're not relatives, Deaf or CODA sitters can be hard to find, expensive, and are often in high demand. Cooperation is key—other hearing parents are in your shoes, after all, so consider setting up a share or part-time situation.

If you want to find a Deaf or CODA caregiver, be ready to network like a motherfucker: reach out to your local deaf school, deaf services agency, Deaf hiking group, Deaf synagogue, and so on. Facebook hard; there's at least one nationwide ASL childcare group online, along with local groups that often serve as job boards for these kinds of requests.[24] Don't overlook teenagers, young adults, and retirees who want to lend a hand; even if they can only do a couple hours a week, a couple of hours of fluent ASL exposure can really add up over time.

Be aware that Deaf caregivers are throwing a lifeline to your family. Deaf adults care deeply about deaf kids and can go out of their way to make sure they get the support they need. That means sitters will sometimes be commuting long distances, struggling through difficult communication with families, or making other compromises to show up for your baby. Be patient and kind, communicate clearly, pay them fairly,[25] and understand that you're getting a gift.

If you can't find a responsible Deaf adult (or tolerably irresponsible Deaf teenager), another option is a hearing interpreting student from a local school or community college. They're often looking for experience with the Deaf community and always looking for cash. Stay away from beginners if you can; you can even reach out to professors and department heads to see if they can do a little matchmaking. While an ASL 3 or 4 student is still years away from mastering the language, they're a lot better than nothing, and getting to that level shows that they're committed to continuing their education, so their skills will hopefully grow along with your child.

Just be careful when hiring a hearing ITP student. It can be tempting to see them as the easier option to work with because they're hearing, or look at them as a 2-for-1 English and ASL package deal, but under no circumstances should you hire an interpreting student *instead* of a fluent Deaf signer.

Childcare Swaps

If you're home with your child or work part-time, another option for finding that care/language/socialization trifecta might be a childcare exchange or swap with a Deaf parent or family where you take turns watching each other's

---

[24]Sites like Care.com sometimes come through, but they don't screen the language skills of applicants, so there's likely to be a lot of "I bet I can sign" people listing ASL as a language. You'll need to really evaluate the skills of any wild hearing nanny you catch this way.

[25]*At least* at the going rate for nannies in your area.

kids. Finding this arrangement can be a major undertaking, but it's potentially free, and free is a very good price. Plus, it can take the burden off of a stay-at-home parent for a couple of hours a week, and that kind of breathing room is literally priceless.

Again, you'll have to scour and post at all the Deaf agencies, schools, and orgs in your area to find a matching family, with the added difficulty that the Deaf parents are likely to have hearing babies, so they won't necessarily be plugged into the same early intervention networks that you're in. This can work to your advantage, though: Deaf families with hearing children are sometimes interested in getting their little CODAs exposure to spoken English, so swapping with your family can be a win / win.

The same cautions about communication and understanding apply as for Deaf sitters. Doing a childcare swap can require a lot of negotiation, trust, and compromise for both families, but spending time with a caring Deaf adult and getting exposed to Deaf family life is priceless.

Evaluating DHH Programs and Schools

Rules of thumb to keep in mind when you're checking out a classroom, whether it's for your infant, toddler, or pre-kindergartener, and whether it's private or run by the state or the district.

Deaf Teachers for Deaf Children

The first question to ask when gauging the quality of a deaf program, from the tiniest preschool upward, is "where are the Deaf professionals?" While there are many wonderful hearing teachers working in deaf education, programs that won't, or can't retain Deaf teachers *in leadership roles,* not just as classroom aides or other assistants, are sus.

Kids need role models. Having Deaf teachers means having someone like them around, an adult who's in charge, who's educated, who can lead and care for other people. It might seem trivial, but deafness is rare enough, and some schools are neglectful enough, that deaf kids can get to adulthood themselves before they meet another Deaf adult. Needless to say, this is a *problem.*

It's not *just* role modeling, though. If there aren't Deaf eyes in the classroom, there's the potential to miss many issues and opportunities. No matter how smart and empathetic a hearing teacher is, they will never have the experience of growing up deaf. The problems deaf kids face can be very subtle; a Deaf teacher who's been there themselves can recognize and address issues a hearing teacher can't see or understand.

And if you're in a signing program, a random hearing teacher may not have the top-level ASL skills you want modeled for your children. Worse than that, the language skills for hearing staff can be *far* below fluent: I was surprised after completing a level-1 ASL course at our local adult-ed program that I qualified to act as a classroom assistant in California. After only three months of night classes, I wasn't qualified to squeegee whiteboards.

In some ways, the lack of Deaf adults in the administration or on the board of a program can be more damaging than a lack of Deaf staff. Without Deaf eyes on hiring and professional supervision, otherwise well-meaning organizations can end up hiring hearing teachers with poor language skills or patronizing attitudes that drag down educational standards. What you'll sometimes see in a mostly hearing program is a process of lock-out, where Deaf staff or teachers struggle to get problems fixed because hearing administrators don't recognize them or don't acknowledge their expertise. These kinds of schools churn through Deaf employees but never retain them long or promote them into supervisory roles.

This doesn't mean every hearing teacher or administrator is bad (or that every Deaf teacher is good!) As I've said, there are many talented hearing folks in deaf education, and you'll find them at all levels from classroom assistant to principal. But the more accomplished a hearing educator is in the field, the more they should understand and advocate for Deaf leadership, and the less eager they should be to take the place of a Deaf professional in the top levels of an organization. Size is a factor, too: sometimes programs are so small or understaffed that getting even one Deaf teacher is a big deal. But even in that situation, you should always ask, "if there's only *one* teacher, why are they *not* Deaf?"

Beware of Cute Babies

Another snare lurking in infant and toddler programs is the fact that children are *adorable*. While that's lucky for us, cuteness can work like a smokescreen to conceal a lot of problems in a bad preschool environment. If you don't know what to look for, a room full of typically developing deaf babies with full language access and great long-term prospects can seem just as sweet—or just as chaotic and messy—as a room full of language-deprived children with years of struggle ahead of them.

Language issues in infants and toddlers can be almost invisible because they are starting at the bottom of a developmental curve. Typical hearing children are expected to be soaking up language for at least a year before they start talking back. And although the average deaf baby can be signing back *sooner* than that, bad teachers round *up* instead of down, and won't even worry about missed milestones until eighteen months or more have passed.

Infant and toddler programs that deprive their babies of language can get away with a lot because the real damage isn't showing up until after everyone graduates. Like a rocket trying to escape the earth's gravity, a baby needs to build up a lot of early momentum. Programs that don't provide children with strong, accessible language models are starving their engines of fuel, but you can't see that until they come crashing back to earth in kindergarten. So don't get distracted by the astronaut's dimples: what's cute and appropriate in a one-year-old is a serious language delay in a three-year-old and a developmental disability in a five-year-old.

One way of controlling for this is to catch up with parents of kids who've been through the program, and not just the "superstar" graduates, either. Now that Oscar is older, we've been able to meet kids who've gone through several of the different early childhood options in our area, and we can see how some programs are setting kids up for success, while others… aren't.

Beware of Low Expectations

Yet another trap. Deafness alone isn't an intellectual disability, but plenty of hearing professionals treat it like one. Bad DHH programs will churn out generations of kids with language delays, behavioral issues, poor academic skills, and other symptoms of language deprivation and don't look at their own bad outcomes because, after all, aren't these part and parcel of deafness? This kind of reflexive audism is everywhere.

For the Deaf Disabled or Deaf + kids, low expectations are even more harmful. These are kids for whom early intervention can be most effective and give them a strong basis for later learning and success, but they are often tracked as either "deaf" or "disabled" and not given appropriate support in both areas. Their deafness can sometimes even get missed because clinicians wrongly assume that language delays somehow come with the territory of their other disabilities, or their deafness is downplayed or sidelined because they have "more urgent" issues, and they end up language deprived on top of everything else. It's always "both and," never "either / or," and this is reflected in the *Individuals with Disabilities Education Act*—districts are required by federal law to help children with *everything* right from the start.

Find Deaf Advice

In general, the local Deaf community will know what's up with schools and programs in your area, which ones are good and which to avoid. The Deaf world is small, the culture values schools and education, and in general, folks are up in each other's business. The average Deaf adult will know a lot more about the different preschool options in their area than the average hearing adult. After all, they're likely to know a graduate, parent, or teacher, or to *be* a graduate of a given program themselves.

This is not a rock-solid *guarantee.* Deaf people are as diverse a group as anyone else, but as a rule, the Deaf community knows which programs work for kids and which ones are disabling, abusive, or weird. These days, thanks to social media, it's easier than ever to find your local people, and it's worth snooping online to get hooked up with your area's Deaf scene.

You can also look for professional help. Contact your local deaf services agency, your local deaf school's outreach center, or your Deaf mentor or coach if you've got one already, and get their perspective. They will typically have a 300-foot view of your nearby services, and even if you think your child won't be a good fit for the deaf school, they are going to have an enormous amount of insight into the local programs and which one will work for them.

One note of caution: while hearing parents of deaf kids[26] are sometimes a good resource, they're often just starting to figure their way through deaf education themselves and won't have the kind of insight that Deaf adults

---

[26]Yeah that's me. *Feel* the hypocrisy.

and professionals do. Often, their recommendations can skew toward those programs that cater more to parents than to the children. Some places put their main efforts into marketing, not teaching—the school with the nicest pamphlet or smoothest outreach person is not necessarily the best place for your child, but they can fool newbies.

Deaf Educational Philosophies

When you're figuring out your options for specialized schools, preschools, and other programs, their deaf-educational philosophy is usually the easiest thing to check. It's generally listed in the "about" or "academics" section of the website, and teachers and administrators will just flat-out tell you; these are foundational to their approach. Mainstream schools, on the other hand, may or may not have these approaches explicitly stated or used in their teaching, which is one of many reasons you'll need to be extra cautious about them.

If you skipped the history chapter (good for you!) just know that deaf-ed philosophies are often presented to parents the old-fashioned way, as either speaking or signing, "oral" or "manual." That actually confuses things. If you go by those labels, you'd think that there would be no English taught in the signing schools and that all signing programs provide essentially the same thing.

The truth is, *all* programs that use ASL also teach English. On the other hand, programs that use sign systems like SEE, PSE, or Cued Speech aren't actually using a sign language; they're presenting only English to their students in different forms, and they sometimes have more in common with speech-only oral programs than with schools using ASL.

It's more useful to think of schools as either *bilingual*, using ASL and English, or *monolingual*, using only English, whether that English is spoken or represented with a sign system. For deaf children of hearing families, bilingual programs can guarantee full language access and are especially important for children still acquiring their first language. Since the consequences of missing the language window are so severe, they're the best choice. Unfortunately, they are the least common option, and there may or may not be one in your area, or even in your state.

Monolingual programs, whether they go all-in on hearing technology and oralism or whether they use some artificial sign system, all carry a higher risk of language deprivation for your child, but given the state of deaf education in the United States, you may not have much of a choice. Deaf kids can succeed in a monolingual program, but you're still working without a net. If you find your kid attending a monolingual program, monitoring your baby's language development and supplementing their education with fluent ASL is going to be a bigger challenge.

Bilingual Philosophies

Bilingual-Bicultural (Bi-Bi or BiBi): The gold standard approach for teaching deaf kids—it's been in practice for about forty years under the Bi-Bi name, but it has roots in the Deaf Renaissance of the nineteenth century and the founding of the American School for the Deaf by Gallaudet and Clerc. It's now common in most state-run day and residential schools for the deaf, and it's essentially the same approach you might see in a foreign language immersion program for French or Mandarin. Bi-Bi uses ASL as the classroom language but teaches English as a subject, with the goal of having kids fluent in both ASL and written English, as well as mastering other aspects of the standard curriculum like math, science, history, social studies, and so on.[27]

For deaf kids of hearing parents, the benefits of this type of program are enormous, especially for young children. Exposure to fluent language models means that infants entering a Bi-Bi program are at much lower risk for language deprivation or language delay. In fact, kids who enter Bi-Bi programs before age three potentially get that cognitive "bilingual bonus" of learning two languages early on, and their long-term academic scores track with same-age hearing children. Since classroom instruction is accessible right from the beginning, the learning opportunities are immediate; they don't have to master

---

[27]For the preschool set, the focus will actually be on pre-literacy and pre-numeracy skills, which are equally important stepping stones to learning. These include vocabulary building, counting, letter and number recognition, and social skills like self-regulation, turn-taking, and so on that they need to get by in kindergarten and beyond.

numbers or letters while also trying to make sense of input from their hearing devices or waste time figuring out how to pronounce "triceratops."

Deaf kids also get enormous social advantages; having a classroom full of signing peers and mentors means that they get to have closer and more meaningful relationships (ever try making a friend through an interpreter?) When my son goes to his Bi-Bi school, there's no missing out, and no dinner table syndrome at his desk. He's not just "the deaf kid"; he's the goofball, he's the math whiz, he's the one obsessed with bats. Every social role and opportunity is open to him, and his childhood is much richer for that.

Bi-Bi schools accept children with all levels of spoken language skills, from kids who only use ASL to children like my son, who mostly uses English outside of class. And while the emphasis in a Bi-Bi program will be on every student being *literate* in English and *fluent* in ASL, that doesn't mean that spoken English isn't taught. Bi-Bi programs will typically have pull-out services, special time and space where children can work on receptive and expressive English skills with SLPs, ToDs, and peers. This comes in addition to outside English support services your kid can get from their home school district.

The "bicultural" aspect of Bi-Bi comes out in the explicit teaching of Deaf history and Deaf cultural values: inviting Deaf storytellers to perform at the school, celebrating important Deaf figures and current events, and connecting with the larger Deaf community. I saw this during my son's first week of preschool here in California. It happened to be career week, and each day they had a speaker attend: a Deaf doctor, a Deaf veterinarian, a CODA firefighter, and a woman training to be the world's first Deaf astronaut. These were all busy people, to say the least, but they took time from their day to talk to *a class of toddlers* and show them that they could achieve anything. This kind of engagement and support by the Deaf community can create opportunities no other kind of school can match.

Other bilingual programs: Sometimes called "Bilingual-Bimodal," "ASL and English Bilingual Education," or similar arrangements, bilingual programs are typically the same or similar to Bi-Bi programs—often it's just a difference in terminology because the average hearing parent doesn't know what the heck a Bi-Bi school is (Sarah Lawrence?). Any program that keeps a classroom separation between signed ASL and spoken English, and that has fluent language models for ASL, is off to a good start.

Beware programs that are using "bilingual" as a synonym for the unfluent mixing of languages, like the Total Communication programs described below. Programs where teachers SimCom or use a sign system like SEE are not bilingual, and programs without strong Deaf leadership are a red flag. That kind of linguistic SlapChop isn't going to help your kid in the long run.

Monolingual Philosophies

Total Communication (TC): It's a shame. Total Communication was a revolution when it first appeared in the late 1960s; just use whatever works to teach deaf kids. Teach with sign language, spoken language, writing, or other communication strategies—go nuts. Even today, TC is presented as the best of both worlds, but hearing teachers and administrators couldn't follow through on its promise. In reality, modern TC has become a marketing term for monolingual programs that don't *technically* forbid sign, but don't actually provide accessible natural language in the form of ASL. By offering an illusion of language access, TC programs share a huge responsibility with oral-only programs in the language deprivation epidemic.

The issue is that TC has no guidelines or official pedagogy. Because there's no standard for fluent language exposure, "whatever works" can quickly become "whatever works for the teachers or administration." In reality, most TC programs have teachers using SimCom SEE or PSE, sometimes with different teachers in the same program using different sign systems at different levels of proficiency. Since SimCom exposes children to oversimplified spoken English and degraded or incomprehensible signing— remember that even teachers with pristine SEE skills are still not signing a natural language—classrooms can end up a mishmash with no strong language models at all.

Some kids can do ok in this environment, but these tend to be the ones whose residual hearing would allow them to do ok in a purely oral program, or who have ASL access at home. Many more kids end up with incomplete language acquisition and language deprivation.

Story time: our local "model DHH preschool" used TC. It was the service provider for our district and within walking distance from our house. At first, it seemed ideal. We spoke to the program director, who was also our itinerant ToD. She was very nice, and the school had great facilities. When we sat in on classes, they spoke and used what looked to us like a sign language at the same time (friends, it was SEE).

But the vibe gave us pause. We asked the few Deaf people we'd met so far; they were not enthusiastic. One of them warned us about SEE. Another said, "Look at the way the kids act in the classroom. They only communicate with the teacher—never with each other." We asked the program director if they taught ASL and got unclear answers ("Oh we have one assistant in the morning who uses it with the babies!"). We took a harder look at their staff: Deaf classroom assistants, a Deaf secretary, Deaf janitors, hearing teachers, hearing administrators, and a hearing board of directors.

We passed.

Note that because of the "anything goes" nature of the TC label, if a classroom practices research-supported bilingual education, having separate times to use English and ASL, and using suitable language models for both languages, that could technically be both "TC" and a good program. Some programs that still fly the TC flag, or have it buried deep in their never-updated "about" pages, are, in practice, bilingual, using ASL and English separately. But if they're SimCom'ing with SEE, PSE, or similar, beware.

Oral programs: listening and spoken language (LSL) and similar: These are the classic "speech-only" approaches to deaf education, focused on using hearing aids or cochlear implants to acquire English. These typically operate under AG Bell's trademark-protected Listening and Spoken Language rubric, which controls the professional-level LSLS certifications for educators. The sole emphasis on spoken English means that these programs are higher risk for language deprivation for deaf children, particularly children who have not already established a strong L1. While they can offer quality English-language instruction and services, LSL-based programs are not better supported by research than generic spoken language interventions, and their blind spots around risk and *iatrogenic*[28] harm make them a bad bet for deaf babies.

---

[28]Injury caused by doctors (or, in this case, teachers).

These programs might use either an Auditory-Verbal Therapy approach or an Auditory Oral one. Auditory Verbal focuses on sound exclusively—ASL, and even speechreading, are forbidden. Auditory Oral is far less common these days: it permits speechreading but still focuses on spoken English as the L1 and language of instruction, and typically forbids using ASL in school. These programs might also discourage children and parents from singing outside of school and generally tie therapy, education, and medical interventions tightly together, creating an environment where speech is the all-encompassing focus. Not only does this put kids at risk of language deprivation, but it can also crowd out other types of education and social learning.

Even for children who have access to spoken language with their devices, learning via prosthetics can require a huge effort and can make the school experience especially stressful. Kids in oral classroom settings often come home exhausted from the long periods of extreme focus required—known in the trade as *listening fatigue*. A competent oral program will take listening fatigue into account and give kids regular breaks from their technology. But just requiring such high levels of concentration from young students goes against what we know about early childhood education, and it makes school a chore and a "session" rather than allowing children to learn through play and natural interaction.

These days, many specialized oral DHH programs are offered only to young children, with the goal of graduating a kid into a mainstream classroom around kindergarten or first grade. Often, oral programs will be aggressive in recruiting newly identified infants and toddlers only to shed them when their language skills aren't progressing and the children are starting to show signs of language deprivation. And because oral schools tend to pass students into the mainstream, kids with an oral education can also hit a wall as they get older, particularly around grades three to five, as lessons and social interactions with hearing teachers and peers become more complex and demanding. Deaf adults who were "oral success stories" often report feeling isolated and depressed, getting good grades only by excessive grinding and after-school catch-up, lacking friends and feeling pressure to hide their struggles from their parents and teachers.

If you find yourself in an area with no other good options, oral programs might help support your child and develop their English skills. Just keep in mind that they can be high-risk, and their baked-in bias against sign language and Deaf culture and identity can do a lot of harm.

Mainstreaming

Beginning with *the Rehabilitation Act of 1973*, neighborhood schools have been open to children with disabilities. With the addition of *IDEA* and the *ADA*, the options for kids to attend public schools have expanded. This is an immense achievement on the part of disabled Americans, including Deaf activists, who fought tooth and nail for both laws to be passed. But deaf kids in particular are often waging an uphill battle in public schools to get the education they're entitled to.

Mainstreaming is now by far the most common form of school for deaf kids in America. In some ways, it's purely a numbers game; although the population of deaf children is small, most states don't have the capacity to teach them all in specialized deaf schools and programs. In the whole of Texas, which has an estimated 7,000 deaf children, there is only one state school serving about 500 kids. Most states are similar—California has only two state schools and two bilingual district schools, and some, like Nebraska or New Hampshire, have no dedicated deaf schools at all.

But when you look inside the system, you'll find that mainstreaming means different things depending on your school district and the age of your child. It could mean a dedicated DHH classroom with only deaf peers, a generic Special Ed class in the local pre-K program with a mix of peers with different disabilities, or it could be placement in a public (or private) classroom alongside only hearing students. In terms of philosophy, school districts tend to lean very monolingual and oral, but there's a lot of variation. For the sake of this chapter, anywhere your child's education is handled directly by a local school district or "normal" private school—overseen by hearing administrators—is a mainstream environment.

Mind the Gap

Your first hurdle in a mainstream environment is going to be the information gap. Hearing teachers and run-of-the-mill special educators—no matter their skill or their good intentions—are starting from very far behind when faced with a deaf child. And even if your child's teachers are knowledgeable teachers of the deaf, or in extraordinary cases, even Deaf ToDs, it is virtually guaranteed their boss, and their boss's boss, know zilch about pediatric deafness, deaf education, language acquisition, ASL curriculum, and so on. Since principals and program directors hold enormous power over what happens in the classroom, this makes their lack of knowledge your kid's problem. And ignorance is kind of a best-case scenario—teachers or administrators with outdated beliefs about deaf ed can make your kid's time in mainstream school a living hell.

You will need to Tiger Mom the shit out of this situation. Show up on day one with the knowledge and willingness to oversee what's happening and intervene when you see something that's not right. Observe your kid in their classroom early and often, and watch how the teachers and assistants interact with your baby. Keep your IFSP/IEP/504 handy and watch if they're fulfilling their end of the bargain. And find Deaf advice and oversight where you can—be it a Deaf mentor or coach, educational advocate, itinerant ToD, or other Deaf professional: literally anyone you can trust to give their outside opinion on your child's progress and skills.

Watch the Attitude

One easy way hearing teachers can screw up the mainstream experience for a deaf kid is to get weird about them; not only is it a depressing burden having a weird teacher, that weirdness will spread from the teacher to the students.

I've already discussed low expectations and patronizing behavior, but well-meaning teachers can also end up focusing too much on a child's hearing status and framing everything in the classroom around what a child can and can't hear. There's a specific ASL sign for AUDISM that really seems to describe this sort of thing, with your hands making a little box around the ear, isolating hearing as the most important part of a person.

Teachers who harp on a deaf kid's hearing and who constantly remind their peers about it can single them out without meaning to. A deaf kid is a *visual* kid. Show, don't tell is the name of the game, and focusing on what they can do and what works for them, rather than on the sound they're not getting, is important.

Social Studies

> At first glance, many deaf people, myself included, are able to make it in the mainstream. We do it with smoke-and-mirrors fake smiles and lots of nodding. Often, we're reinforced by well-meaning parents and teachers who gush over how well we appear to assimilate. They're thrilled if we learn our ABCs, but oblivious to the social isolation we deal with.
>
> Mark Drolsbaugh, Deaf author, from *Madness in the Mainstream*

The next question to answer about a mainstream environment is, "how will my kid make friends?" Baby friends are easy—parallel play doesn't require a lot of chatting—but as your child makes the developmental climb from infant to toddler to kindergartener, more and more language comes in.

Sometimes this can work to your kid's advantage. Some deaf folks value their hearing friends from childhood and have cousins, classmates, or next-door neighbors who learned ASL alongside them, or have other homegrown, time-tested communication strategies. But while it can be easy to get sentimental about childhood friendships, remember that kids swing both ways. While they can sometimes jump social gaps that scare adults, they can also single out other children for trivial differences. Bullying is very common for mainstreamed kids, as is plain isolation, where a deaf child is locked out of the social life of the classroom.

Good teachers will be mindful of this, but again, hearing teachers can miss a lot of the exclusion and struggle that deaf children, even the ones who exclusively use spoken English, can experience in a hearing environment. The presence of other DHH kids in the classroom is a good start. It's a common experience for parents to have their mainstream kid "do OK," but suddenly go through a transformation when placed in a Deaf environment. Kids who seemed to be loners, bookworms, or who had just one or two besties are suddenly social butterflies, spreading their wings in a place where communication is straightforward.

Mainstream Flavors

The hearing classroom. Aka, "mainstreaming classic." This is a deaf student in a hearing classroom with hearing peers and a hearing teacher, and whatever accommodations your child needs—an ASL interpreter, an FM or Rogers system, visits from the ToD, and so on. This can work for some kids in some ways, but you'll need to keep a sharp eye out for the social and educational pitfalls listed above.

Special education / resource room: Beware the OmniSpEd! Potentially mainstreaming at its worst. While some kids need the support a special ed classroom can provide, districts sometimes take a one-size-fits-all approach and shunt deaf student into special education environments alongside children with many different needs. No matter how skilled a special education teacher is in their area of expertise, a heart surgeon is not a rocket scientist, and a "vanilla" SpEd teacher is not a ToD.

This caution also applies to Deaf + and Deaf Disabled children. A deaf child with an additional disability needs language access and deaf-ed expertise, full stop, and no school system should be throwing hearing and deaf students together solely on the basis of their "other" diagnosis. It's unfair to the children, it's unfair to the educators, and it's also a clear violation of IDEA, which explicitly states that children with disabilities will get services tailored to their specific circumstances. Especially in a classroom setting where a hearing teacher, trained in teaching hearing kids, is trying to teach both hearing and deaf students, someone—the deaf one—is going to get shortchanged.

This doesn't mean it's always inappropriate to place a deaf child in a special ed program—it's really dependent on what services and expertise your kid needs access to—but any district that uses SpEd as the default needs a hard look, and isn't necessarily going to be scrupulous about holding your child to appropriate standards or adjusting their services as they develop.

TC in the mainstream. Because there's no rule book, Total Communication is a very popular format in mainstream programs. Any program that incorporates any amount of sign, no matter how inept or insufficient, can claim to be Total Communication, so this makes it easy for school districts to set up TC classrooms and, uh, "serve everyone." Hearing teachers using SEE are still the most common type of signing ToD out there, and plenty of administrators don't know the difference between a well-meaning hearing SEE signer and an ASL-fluent Deaf signer. Some even *prefer* hearing teachers because they're considered easier for the administrators and parents to communicate with, no matter the consequences for students. Nuts to all this.

Bilingual in the mainstream. On the other hand, a good bilingual program can be a godsend if you're far away from the state-run deaf schools. They can be as simple as a separate DHH room in a school or pre-K setting with a few students and a signing teacher and aide—as long as there are fluent adults modeling ASL for the kids for most of the school day, these can be successful for deaf kids, especially if they gather enough of them together. A critical mass of six or eight children, even if they're spread across a few grades, can become a self-sustaining peer group that supports strong social and linguistic skills.

Unfortunately, these sorts of classrooms can be a moving target. Small bilingual programs can wink in and out of existence frequently because of the low numbers of deaf children and qualified teachers, and the whims of hearing school administrators. Often, a good program will be sustained by one or two ASL-fluent teachers in isolation, and when they leave, the classroom ends up going downhill, changing to an oral or signing system method, or just closing. Or, the teacher in the next grade up will be a mediocre SEE-signer or hardcore oralist! This can create a hazardous situation for kids, where an environment that was supportive and successful for them turns into something else over the summer. If you find yourself in a bilingual mainstream program, keep an eye on the staff at all grade levels, and be ready to advocate hard for your kid and their teachers.

Language Learning in the Mainstream (Interpreters Don't Cut It)

In situations where your child is immersed in an English-language classroom, your first concern is fluent language exposure. If you want to build your child's ASL skills, it's not enough to just have a classroom interpreter. Why?

Interpreting is a specialized skill, both for the terp and for the kid using a terp, and the process is very far from natural language immersion. Interpreters are required to stay by their client's side and interpret all the English-language conversation around them, acting as a conduit for language to and from teachers and peers—the interactions are all indirect. Because of this, there's very little of the natural give and take that happens in regular conversation, and research has demonstrated that, even if a child has skillful interpreters, they will often struggle to fully acquire ASL from those indirect interactions alone.

The sad part of this is that while there are many skilled educational interpreters out there, your school district might not have strong standards or oversight for terps. If you're a hearing parent, it can take a long time to figure out if a terp is good or not, and districts are usually not in any rush to replace filled positions. If your kid needs ASL and is in any kind of mainstream program, terps are important, but not sufficient.

Safeguards and Allies for Mainstream Kids

IFSP and IEP plans offer you some legal protection against a bad mainstream environment, but not much. Even if you're able to get appropriate goals and accommodations written into the plan, without top-to-bottom competence, from the classroom assistants up to the principal, the plan might never get implemented properly, or erode as the school year goes on, leaving your kid stranded. Young children usually can't articulate problems and communication breakdowns except by acting out in various ways, so issues can go unaddressed for weeks or months, or get blamed on your kid's behavior, which is ass-backwards but common.

Once you discover a problem, immediately contact the teachers and be prepared to call a full IEP meeting. If your school agrees to fix it—and that's a big if—it may take more time to make it right. Meanwhile, your child will be missing out on irreplaceable language development and learning, so act fast.

Also know that a teacher can follow an IEP to the letter and still give your child next to nothing for their education. Ultimately, there's no piece of paper on earth, barring one with a dead president on it, that will get a burnt-out, disinterested, or hostile teacher to approach your child with the mix of empathy, curiosity, and enthusiasm that good teaching needs. Running through the motions is never enough.

504 plans are to IEPs as Saran Wrap is to a Trojan. If something isn't right about how the teacher, aides, or technology is working, the most you're typically allowed is a discussion with the principal or another authority figure. If appeals through the school's process don't make it right, you will need to contact your local Office of Civil Rights in order to file a complaint / lawsuit. Unless your child has *very* few needs, forget it.

Itinerant teachers of the deaf: When your child's primary instructor isn't a deaf ed'ster, itinerant ToDs might be offered as backstops. These teachers come to class to observe and do *push-in* (in-class) or *pull-out* (outside class) sessions and assessments with your child. While these itinerants might have some impact, districts will often offer pitiful itinerant face time for deaf kids, giving them things like fifteen minutes of instruction per month.

Even if your kid's ToD is able to successfully monitor your child's education, they may not have any influence over what happens during most of your child's day. Regardless of their expertise, itinerants may not be able to get teachers and aides to cooperate or move the needle on the district's bad decisions—they're potentially an ally with little power.

Educational audiologists: Your district Ed.AuD should be keeping an eye on your kid's progress and pointing out any potential traps—situations where their hearing devices aren't going to be effective, behaviors that indicate they're missing classroom discussions or instructions. Like an itinerant ToD, a clued-in audiologist is better than a clueless one, but an Ed.Aud may have limited power over your kid's overall experience.

Educational interpreter: A good educational interpreter can make a big difference in a deaf kid's mainstream experience and are often the make-or-break support for kids in hearing classrooms. But like itinerant ToDs, even if they are compassionate and skillful, they sometimes work at a major disadvantage. Unlike the real world, where professional 'terps work in pairs for long assignments, in a classroom setting, an interpreter is often working alone for hours at a stretch. They may have unreasonable expectations placed on them to "manage" the classroom or their child in ways that interfere with interpretation, and they often do not get the respect of teachers or classroom assistants and have little influence on their behavior. And a bad terp, well . . .

Bad Allies

When you're in a mainstream program and draw a *bad* ToD, educational interpreter, audiologist, and so on, this can be a massive problem for your kid. A 'terp or ToD with substandard language skills (or just bad professional practice) will end up creating a lot of gaps in your child's education, and then covering up or excusing them in IEP meetings to cover their own ass, and a bad audiologist can be a major obstacle to getting your child-appropriate services—"Well he can hear all the Ling 6 during our sessions . . ."

Teachers, administrators, and LEAs with no deaf-ed experience will reflexively look to these folks for guidance, potentially complicating IEP meetings. And because there is a shortage of all kinds of staff in American schools, along with strong employment protections in many school districts, they can be difficult or impossible to fire or reassign. See *Dealing with Bad Professionals* for more on giving them the ax.

Educational Interpreters under IFSP, IEP, and 504 Plans

Educational ASL interpreters are an area where parents often get into conflict with their school district. Good interpreters are hard to find and are a big expense for the district, so it's common for districts to fight interpreters requested under an IFSP / IEP / 504—and it's just as common for them to supply poorly trained or otherwise substandard terps.

This is illegal: your child almost always has the right to a quality interpreter. While IDEA or Section 504 may or may not require an interpreter depending on the district's own reading of the law, the Americans with Disabilities Act (ADA) is *very clear* and states that in all public schools, the "primary consideration" for accommodations falls to the party with the disability. And while IDEA is the law that covers most aspects of special education, *schools must always also follow the ADA.*

That means that, regardless of whether the district considers the particular accommodations and therapies they've supplied to your kid sufficient, you and your child get primary consideration in deciding how they can *access communication in the classroom*, and that the level of communication has to be *equal to their peers*. Even if they are refusing all other ASL-related services, they will still be in violation of the ADA if they don't give you an interpreter if you ask for one.

The Federal Department of Education has issued guidance to this effect, and you should use it. I link to this document at willfertman.com, but you can just

Google *Frequently Asked Questions on Effective Communication for Students with Hearing, Vision, or Speech Disabilities in Public Elementary and Secondary Schools;* check out section 10 in particular. And while you will still need to exhaust your IDEA appeals process before you can use Title II, your district will be on the hook for monetary damages to your child for every minute of class time they miss. Remind them of that when you start the process.

School Placement, FAPE, and the Problem with LRE

One term you'll run into a lot in IFSPs and IEPs when talking about placement—where your child goes to school—is *free and appropriate public education* (FAPE). That's shorthand for your child's right to an education under federal law. All school districts in the United States must provide FAPE for all their students, regardless of their disability. If your district can't offer FAPE in your neighborhood school, they need to pay to send your child to another public, state, or private school or program. That's the *free* part.

The *appropriate* part is harder to pin down because it varies depending on a child's individual needs. To help determine what's appropriate for each kid, IDEA says that education must occur in the *least restrictive environment* (LRE). This creates a little chain of logic to follow: for a school or program to be FAPE for your baby, it must also be the LRE for your baby. It's a standard that's helped students with many different disabilities access education through the years, but when districts thoughtlessly apply LRE to deaf children, it can lead to disaster.

IDEA was written in 1975, with school desegregation very much on everyone's mind. "Separate but equal" schools had been recognized as inherently unjust for students of color just two decades before, and so IDEA emphasized the same solution, placing disabled kids into mainstream public schools as a fundamental way to ensure their rights:

> To the maximum extent appropriate, children with disabilities . . . are educated with children who are not disabled, and special classes, separate schooling, or other removal of children with disabilities from the regular

educational environment occurs only when the nature or severity of the disability of a child is such that education in regular classes . . . cannot be achieved satisfactorily.

"To the maximum extent" means that districts will often bend over backwards to keep kids at local public schools no matter what kind of a shit sandwich it is for your kid, sometimes torturing the letter of the law to fit their view of what is appropriate.

If you disagree with your child's mainstream placement, and your state isn't a "school choice" state, the burden will be on you to prove that the school *isn't* the LRE for your kid. You may need to lobby your district, go into mediation, file a complaint with the State educational agency, or get an administrative hearing under due process in order to get your child placed in a better classroom. It can take years of your time and gallons of your blood.[29]

Young deaf children who don't have a first language are particularly hurt by a "mainstream-first" interpretation of LRE—they're literally disabled through language deprivation in hearing classrooms, waiting until they fall far enough behind to "qualify" for a deaf school or other program. But even kids with strong spoken English skills can find themselves extremely restricted by a typical public school. Accommodations like FM systems or ASL interpreters often don't cover the entire school day, or even all their class time, and don't help with incidental learning or the important social interactions kids have with their peers. Hearing the words spoken by the teacher is only a small part of the school experience; if it's the only part that works, sometimes at great effort, kids are missing out. Deaf adults, even "oral success stories" who have strong spoken English and good academic records, often report that mainstream school was isolating, stressful, and unhappy.

For a deaf kid, the least restrictive environment, and the one that gives them the most "mainstream" experience, is often the state deaf school. In a bilingual ASL classroom, deaf children have 100 percent access to language all the time and aren't dependent on kludgy technology or inconsistent hearing

---

[29]Whatever the final outcome, your kid doesn't get those years back. If your district won't permit the placement that's best for your child, and if it's possible for your family, I strongly recommend moving or switching to a more accommodating district. Don't fight—run.

teachers or interpreters for their education. Beyond that, they have full access to social lives, role models, and incidental learning. Any problems they face can be addressed by teachers and staff who have a deep understanding and experience with deaf child development. To steal a line from Chuck E. Cheese, it's where a kid can be a kid.

The federal government actually understands this. In a position paper on IDEA from way back in 1992, they tell local districts that they're getting it wrong on LRE for deaf kids:

> The Secretary is concerned that some public agencies have misapplied the LRE provision by presuming that placements in or closer to the regular classroom are required for children who are deaf . . . the regular classroom is an appropriate placement for some children who are deaf, but for others it is not. The decision as to what placement will provide FAPE for an individual deaf child . . . must be made only after a full and complete IEP has been developed that addresses the full range of the child's needs.
>
> Deaf Students Education Services, US Dept. of Education 1992

This should have cleared things up way back when, but the problems continue: for many districts, LRE = mainstream unless proven otherwise.

Tough Love versus Enough Love—Avoiding the Moonshot Mentality

When I talk to parents about mainstreaming versus deaf schools and classrooms, I sometimes get this argument: "The world is hearing. My baby will need to get by with hearing people; why shouldn't they go to a mainstream school to have that experience firsthand?"

The worry is real. Your child will need to learn how to get by in hearing spaces with appropriate accommodations, and also manage situations where they *don't* have the accommodations or access they are due by law. Trusting children to overcome obstacles by themselves is a big and important part of parenting; especially with a deaf kid, there are a lot of moments where letting them figure it all out on their own is the right move. But trying to toughen a kid up by putting them in a position where they are so often isolated and misunderstood, especially when they are very young, can have the opposite effect.

> One of the reasons why I am SO hardcore about even unilateral loss kids getting ASL is simple: there are some parents who think that their kid is automatically going to be on the fast track for a competitive career because they *weren't* given specialized techniques and experiences.
>
> It's very common for kids who were raised with minimal accommodations to struggle socially, and social skills are VITAL to getting a job. If it's hard for a hearing kid to get hired, it's going to be VERY hard for a deaf/hoh kid who was raised in this way—they might not even have gone to deaf camp or had interventions more complicated than an FM or front-row seating.
>
> It's far better to be proactive and give your kid a variety of experiences and techniques so that all bases will be covered. This or that could give your kid wings for their development.
>
> Torrie, Deaf adult

Don't idealize difficulty for your child—*A Boy Named Sue* is just a song. Deaf life is already life in hard mode, and your child needs time and space to develop their skills. That's what school is supposed to be—a place filled with second chances, with cheerleaders on the sidelines and cushions when you fall. Kids become tough and resourceful when they can try things and at least have a shot at succeeding.

Interpreters: Hiring and Firing

For kids and adults who mostly use ASL, interpreters are an essential aspect of getting access to the hearing world. While there are plenty of other ways Deaf folks communicate, a skillful sign language interpreter is often the most direct and unambiguous method. It's also a right guaranteed by American law; nearly every government office and business that serves the public, excluding places of worship, is required to supply an interpreter for your child *at their expense*. This includes your child's doctors and therapists, their school (no matter what your kid's IEP says), the YMCA, and your local Build-a-Bear.

Early and Often

For school or medical appointments, check with the front desk at least a month in advance to make sure that the interpreter booking is in their calendar and that they've actually found a terp. If it's a medical office, make sure that it's written into your kid's chart—even if they're an infant—so there will always be one present when you make an appointment. School districts, hospital systems, or big businesses like Legoland will have ADA offices and contracts with interpreting agencies that make the process pretty straightforward—but make sure they're not just throwing an iPad at you (see *What About Video Relay Interpreting (VRI?)* below).

Any organization smaller than that which doesn't specifically deal with deaf or disabled clients will generally have *no idea* how to order an interpreter. Often, they will say they don't have to, but that's generally bullshit. They are required by law in almost all cases. But while it is their legal responsibility to find a terp for you, for the sake of actually getting someone in the door, I recommend bringing a list of multiple agencies or freelancers that they can contact.

No Terp? Big Problem

Giving enough time, some leads, and making sure they follow through is important because it's almost impossible to get an interpreter on short notice. If you show up to an appointment and they're not there, ditch. Tell the doctor and the secretary that you'll reschedule, and don't compromise. We've canceled multiple checkups when no interpreter appeared; allowing it to slide when the office had plenty of time to make arrangements doesn't hold them accountable, and subjecting our son to something like an exam or procedure without full language access is a non-starter:

> I don't want to bring my child to a checkup where a doctor might touch their body, and they don't have any agency or understanding of what happened. They may come home and assume that it's always ok for adults to touch them like that.
>
> my wife

Walking out—and letting your kid know why—also sets a strong example for them. Children should expect full inclusion and transparent communication from the professionals they interact with, because as they get older and more independent, the stakes for interpreting get higher. In medical and legal settings, competent interpreting is all-important; the Deaf community is filled with stories about communication breakdowns that cost people their health, their freedom, and their lives. Rescheduling a dental cleaning, even if you could have muddled through, shows your kid that you value their agency and models how they should react when someone tries to take it away.

Of course, if it's an emergency, you may have to settle for VRI or do the interpreting yourself, but otherwise there should be no question about the presence of an interpreter. And if you get stood up repeatedly, or if they outright refuse to provide an interpreter, contact your local deaf services agency or disability rights group. You're on your way to a lawsuit.

Playing Favorites

Use them enough, and you'll soon find out which interpreters are a good fit for your kid. It's a question of skill *and* personality—particularly for children, a really good interpreter is going to match your child's energy, keeping them engaged and communication flowing. Get their business cards, and don't be shy about asking for terps by name from an agency, or asking to *not* be assigned particular interpreters who don't gel with your baby.

Bad Terps

Beyond just not being a "kid person," there are some distinct issues to watch out for when an interpreter is working with your child:

SimComming when it's not requested or needed—this will only degrade the quality of their ASL.

Only interpreting direct questions to your child—interpreters should be giving your kid access to *all* conversations in the room.

Getting chatty—terps need to make judgment calls about how much side conversation they'll engage in. Young kids won't expect an interpreter to be robotic language relays, but being too friendly with you or your child can interfere with the job.

Oversimplifying ASL—a skilled interpreter will find age-appropriate, conceptually correct ways to express ideas without losing essential meaning.

Impatience with typical kid behaviors, including tantrums and mischief—even a grouchy or misbehaving child has the right to communication access; they need it *more* than a calm and well-behaved kid.

Commenting on your child's hearing, their devices, ASL skills, speech skills, or other "Deaf stuff"—just no. Silent judgment only.

Telling tales out of school—interpreters have strict rules about client privacy. If it comes out that your terp has been gossiping about you, or if they gossip about other clients *to* you, that's instant death.

Poor skills in general—whether they don't know specific terminology, or they can't follow your child's signing, or if they create any communication barriers, out the door they go.

If you have a bad experience with an interpreter, don't hesitate to file a complaint with the agency you hired them through, or with the Registry of Interpreters for the Deaf (RID) if they are RID-certified.

Interpreter FAQ

Can I Interpret for My Child?

You *can*, but unless it's a quick or impromptu visit it's not a good idea. You'll do it a lot at the ice cream shop, but balancing the role of parent and interpreter can be very challenging in places like a doctor's office. Like SimCom, you're basically trying to speak two languages at once. Having a professional around means you can focus on parenting your child: answering their questions, giving guidance and assurance, and being present mentally and emotionally.

How Do I Order an Interpreter?

If you're making the booking yourself, or if you need to give leads to a business, start by asking your local deaf services agency and the folks in the community for agency recommendations. Different agencies will have different methods—email, online forms, or phone calls (!!!) When you hire an interpreter, they will generally ask you who they'll be interpreting for and what the event is. If you have any preferred terps who work at the agency, let them know.

When Do I Start Booking Interpreters for My Child?

ASAP. We started requesting interpreters for medical appointments when Oscar was an infant; after all, hearing kids have access to language at that age, too. Not only does it normalize having an interpreter present for your child, but it lowers the stakes as you get the hang of the process.

How Much Does Interpreting Cost?

It ain't cheap. Interpreters are professionals, and they're paid professional wages. Although the prices will depend on your area, they can be a hundred dollars an hour or more, and sessions longer than an hour may actually require two interpreters to switch off. For a medical office or school district, this is squarely their problem, and you should never think twice about it.

For small businesses and nonprofit / volunteer orgs, these prices can be very steep, but it does *not* mean your child does not have the right to a terp. Tax rebates are available for providing interpreters, and interpreters will sometimes donate services to various nonprofits or community groups—your local deaf services agency can give them information on this.

One good strategy for low-budget outfits is to get all the deaf kids together with a single interpreter for an event, class, or performance. A dozen guaranteed ticket sales can make the cost of interpreting bearable for a small organization, and it will also help them prepare so you get a better, more accessible experience. Going with friends is more fun anyway!

The high cost and high professional expectations for interpreters mean that when you're hiring one yourself, don't be shy about asking for exactly who and what you need. Although finding, say, a culturally competent interpreter for a South Indian Hindu wedding might be a needle in a haystack, it's worth looking for someone who knows their way around the ceremony.

What's the Deal with Certified Deaf Interpreters (CDIs?)

CDIs are highly skilled Deaf professionals hired to provide interpretation with native fluency and high-level Deaf cultural competence. They generally work in teams with a skilled hearing interpreter providing the "first draft" interpretation, taking what they get from the hearing terp and polishing it into crystal-clear ASL. They are often the best choice for impeccable communication in high-stakes situations like emergency broadcasts, business negotiations, complex medical treatments, and legal cases, but are fairly rare and even more expensive than a plain Jane hearing interpreter.

What about Video Relay Interpreting (VRI)?

VRI is a workaround where the terp appears on a phone, computer, or tablet, Max Headroom-style. While this type of service can be useful for adults, this isn't a good solution for a child.

Using an interpreter is a skill all its own; to master it, kids need plenty of in-person practice with a terp who knows how to express ideas clearly and who can read the whole environment to ensure that critical information is getting passed along. VRI isolates the terp—they can only see and hear a tiny slice of what's happening—and it shrinks them down into a set of hands and a face on a computer screen. For a distractible, possibly upset child, this can make them impossible to understand. The National Association of the Deaf recommends children have in-person terps whenever possible, and they have advocacy letters on their website you can present to businesses that try to foist an iPad off on your kid.

On top of this, VRI is notorious for bad connections, especially in places like hospitals, where a weak Wi-Fi signal will make communication impossible. The random nature of VRI work assignments also means your child can be paired with less skillful terps who don't know the proper lingo and can't clarify concepts. If you're ever using a VRI interpreter and they're not doing an adequate job, you can request a switch on the fly—just say, "I'd like to switch interpreters," and they'll reassign the video feed to another on-shift terp in a second or two. We've done that at least once mid-parent-teacher conference, and it's saved us from some serious misunderstandings.

Medical Issues

Most of this book, I've ignored the doctors. This is deliberate: like I said at the beginning of Part 2, what happens when the doctors aren't around is really the most important part of raising a deaf kid.

Anyways, *I'm* not a doctor and I can't advise you on medical questions. But in my experience as the parent of a deaf child, a big part of your job will be separating what's necessary for your child's health from all the weird biases medical professionals bring to deaf babies. A lot of decisions will be presented to you as medical things when they are really developmental, social, and educational things.

One useful way to sort through these decisions is with the *social model of disability*. The idea is that a difference is only a disability when it stands in the way of what you want or need. Using a wheelchair may not have any impact on your poker game, but being skinny can really hold back your sumo career. Redheads like me need accommodations to live in California and avoid sunburn (or worse), but being short and nearsighted is practically the qualifying exam for becoming a Navy submariner.

Likewise, deafness can be a disability under specific circumstances, but it's not a wound, and it doesn't need healing. Whatever prosthetics or accommodations your child ends up using, the goal of those interventions is to get your kid across their own personal finish lines—ace the test, make a friend, fix their bike, destroy Mars, whatever. When you're making decisions about your child's body, those are the guiding lights to follow, and no surgeon, SLP, or audiologist is going to be there with you or with your child when it all goes down.

Audiograms and the "Hearing Loss" Diagnosis

When you get your kid's hearing tested—whether it's an ABR test on a sleeping baby or booth testing on an older kid—the result will be presented to you as an audiogram: a graph of different frequencies of sound and how loud those sounds need to be before your child can actually hear them. It looks like a grid with a bunch of connected dots; pitches move from low on the right to high on the left, and the height of each mark shows the volume your child can detect. X is the left ear, O is the right ear. **Your audiologist should walk you through how to read it, and you should insist that they do.**

Putting together a thorough audiogram can take a long time. My son had at least three ABR tests before the full extent of his deafness was confirmed, so even though he was caught in the newborn screening in the hospital, he didn't have a medical diagnosis of *profound bilateral sensorineural deafness* until he was three months old. This was actually incredibly fast, mostly because he was very, very deaf. The audiologist was like, "I just landed a 747 on his head in stereo, and he's still asleep. We're done here."

Babies with more residual hearing, with progressive hearing loss, or with fluctuating hearing can often take months longer to pin down, and some kids are just wiggle worms who don't cooperate in various ways. This can be a big problem, and it's compounded when the audiologist's office can't schedule, or the insurance company won't pay for, successive tests quickly enough. Getting stuck waiting for the diagnosis means you can't get admitted to Early Intervention, and the sooner you start EI, the better off your kid will be.

If you're spinning your wheels right now, go to your state's Early Intervention website and follow the instructions for *self-referral* to get started immediately. You don't necessarily need a note from a doctor or a complete audiogram to start services. And if you *do* need a note from your audiologist, have a conversation with them and let them know that you need to get your kid referred as soon as possible, *even if testing isn't finished*. Depending on the situation, your audiologist may not have to probe every last frequency. Remember that many audiologists don't have a strong background in language development, so they often don't really understand the impact of a months-long delay could have on an infant, or that going forward with a "good enough" diagnosis won't hurt while you continue to work out the kinks in their 'gram.

The Speech Banana and the Ling 6

Audiological testing spans tones from super-high pitch mosquito buzz all the way down to super-low elephant fart rumbles, but this is a much wider set of frequencies than human voices actually make. Those vocal tones hover around the *speech banana*, a curved zone in the middle of an audiogram that they usually color yellow. Kids who can't hear frequencies that fall into the speech banana won't hear human voices. So while *environmental hearing*—car engines, barking dogs, slappin' bass solos—can be important, most of the focus in pediatric audiology is going to be on accessing sounds in the speech banana.

The Ling 6 sounds are a quick and dirty way to see if your kid can hear those speech banana frequencies without using testing equipment. The human voice tends to make *ah, ooo, eee, sh, sss,* and *mmm* sounds at certain frequencies: if your kid can't hear "ah," that means they're likely not hearing mid-range sounds around 500 Hz. If they can't hear "sss," that means they're probably not picking up high-pitch sounds around 4500 Hz, and so on. Audiologists have standard symbols for the Ling 6, snakes, and airplanes and such, so that they can test your pre-verbal children by having them point to or play with a toy that represents that sound when they hear it. You can also test your kid at home with the Ling 6 to see if their devices are giving them access to these sounds, which is useful.

In general, though, a much bigger deal is made of the Ling 6 than it deserves. Individual tones are not language, and the Ling 6 doesn't even cover the full frequency range of typical speech—it's just a spot-check. A kid can hear and identify the Ling 6 and still not be able to detect or decode speech for a million reasons. So beware of audiologists and speech pathologists who make hearing Ling 6 sounds the be-all and end-all of their work. If you see the Ling 6 popping up in your kid's IFSP or IEP goals, make sure that you have strong functional language goals there as well.

Health Concerns and Medical Testing

In a lot of ways, it doesn't really matter why your baby is deaf, but there are a couple of areas where deafness might be a sign of other health problems, either now or down the road. Doctors will generally have clear guidelines when a child is first identified to screen for these conditions, but American healthcare being what it is, those tests don't always get done, or the results aren't shared with parents very clearly. So if you've got a deaf baby with no other diagnosis, talk with your doctor about the following two issues:

A screening for congenital cytomegalovirus (CMV): this is the most common non-genetic cause of deafness in infants. Infection with the virus while still in the womb can trigger progressive hearing loss in young children and potentially other health problems, including progressive vision loss, motor, and developmental delays. While there are more well-known illnesses that cause congenital deafness, CMV kind of flies under the radar, even among some doctors, but it's very common and mild in everyone except infants; most people don't know they have it. Testing a child for CMV can be tricky. You need a sample of blood that was taken within three weeks of birth,[30] but if you do find it, antiviral treatments might be appropriate to head off future problems.

A genetic test for deaf-linked conditions: most genetic forms of deafness are *non-syndromic*, meaning they only affect hearing, but about one in five kids who inherit their deafness have a *syndromic* form of deafness that can affect their health in other ways. In the old days, when genetic testing was cutting-edge, they would often only test for one or two common genes. Current technology can handle dozens more, so make sure the screening is for a broad spectrum of different mutations. There are specific health considerations for kids with syndromic deafness, ranging from mild to serious, and knowing sooner is always better. Genetic testing can be expensive and may take several months, but it's worth fighting with the insurance company for this one.

More on Genetics—"To Me, My X-Men!"

Half of all deaf children inherit the trait from their parents, but nearly all parents of deaf kids are hearing. Welcome to the screwy world of human heredity!

If you learned about genetics in high school biology class, you might be in for a surprise when you dig into the particulars of different deaf genes: there are nuances here that go way beyond "dominant" and "recessive" that affect how genes are passed on and how they end up expressed in your child's

---

[30] Your baby's dried blood spot (DBS), which is usually collected by the hospital at birth, can be a source of blood for a CMV test.

body. Because it's so variable, it's best to ask your doctor, genetics counselor, or Magneto the Master of Magnetism to explain what's happening in your family's particular case.

In general, though, non-syndromic deaf genes are mutations that cause some level of deafness, but nothing else. They generally have codenames like EYA4 or MYO3A, which describe proteins that the particular gene actually makes in your body. You can find the list on Wikipedia—they're always turning up more. My kid has the most common non-syndromic mutation: GJB2, also known as *connexin-26*. Even though non-syndromic genes don't come with extra health concerns, getting to know your child's particular mutation can help you understand how they can pass from parent to child. This is useful if you want to prepare for possible deaf siblings (or grandkids!)

Syndromic deafness is caused by genes that have impacts on other parts of your child's body and are often named after the doctors who first identified them. Some can be identified just by their symptoms, but others, like Usher or Pendred, aren't always obvious at birth, which is why genetic testing is a good idea. Kids with Usher, for instance, typically lose their vision as they age. Knowing ahead of time can help manage that process and gives you the opportunity to help your child develop DeafBlind life skills like orientation and mobility, Braille literacy, ProTactile sign, and so on. On the other hand, kids with Pendred can easily damage their residual hearing through trauma— no headbutt contests for them—and they might also need to monitor their thyroid hormone levels as they get older. Other syndromes associated with deafness include Down syndrome, Waardenburg, CHARGE, Ehlers-Danlos, Treacher Collins, and dozens more, each with their own set of symptoms and health implications.

Because of the rare nature of many syndromic conditions, and the wide range of effects they have on your child, making connections is even more critical, both with parents of children with the same syndrome and with adults who have the syndrome. There will be information you can only get from other folks in the community, from medical tips or insights into your child's behavior or experience to hints and mentorship that can help your kid live their best life. The Internet is a godsend.

Gene Therapy

As of this writing, there are a few experimental gene therapies for different forms of deafness in testing stages. There will be more in the coming years, and the ones we hear about will likely be effective, to one degree or another, in giving deaf children more access to sound.

So far, the press has treated these therapies uncritically. But just reading the actual scientific papers, I can see similar claims being made about gene therapies that are made about cochlear implants: treatments that seem to be partial, that apply to small numbers of children, and that may not be risk-free, are being presented uncritically as a "cure for deafness."

There are still decades of work to be done in the field, but the need for deeper ethical reasoning is clear. It's not wrong to want your child to hear more, but deafness isn't a disease and no child *needs* these particular treatments. Unfortunately, the emerging gene therapy industry seems to be gearing up to present another charm offensive that may leave many parents disappointed and many children language-deprived. If you are going to enroll your child in a gene therapy program, you're going to want to support their language development with something a lot more reliable—a natural signed language.

Non-Genetic Deafness

Roughly half of deaf babies are deaf because of environmental factors like illness or injury. The most common cause in newborns is an infection before birth with CMV or any of the other charmingly named TORCH[31] pathogens: toxoplasmosis, rubella, cytomegalovirus, herpes, and syphilis. Birth trauma is also a common cause of deafness, especially premature birth and low birth weight. Kids with cerebral palsy are also more likely to be deaf. Later on, deafness can also be caused throughout childhood by complications from ear infections, different forms of meningitis, or as a side effect of antibiotics, chemotherapy, or other medical treatments. The list is endless.

---

[31] The "O" actually stands for Other infections: HIV, syphilis, fifth disease, chickenpox, and Zika. I guess THSFCZRCH wasn't as easy to remember.

Managing Medical Conditions and Medical Trauma

> When my son was born, it was just like, "Can he breathe? Can he eat? Breathe. Eat. Breathe. Eat. Breathe. Eat. It was all urgent and life-threatening, I didn't think about his deafness for months."
>
> Jennifer, hearing parent

Our babies are fragile and tough creatures. Caring for a sick or medically complex child can open you like a knife, and the news that your kid is also deaf can be a real kick in the ass coming at the tail end of a medical crisis or slow-rolling series of issues. This is another area where Deaf mentors and role models can help—finding adults who've gone through your child's challenges or experienced similar things can point you toward the future.

Parents whose deaf kids have ongoing medical conditions are fighting a multifront war and need more than what's in this book; however, there are some essential points to emphasize:

- Don't let doctors neglect deafness in favor of other elements of your child's disability
- If you have a partner, make a plan for how you'll make medical decisions, and share the medical treatment chores where you can—see the chapter *Parents and Partners*
- Be aware of your treatment team's attitude; you want doctors just as empathetic and involved as a kindergarten teacher
- Find professional help where you can: group support, one-on-one counseling, psychiatric medication, and pastoral support can all help get you through
- Patient advocates are gold when you can find them, but you will also need to be ready to advocate for your child yourself

And if your kid is still undergoing medical treatment, you have the right to protect yourself and demand that medical personnel read your child's file before asking you to recite your kid's conditions and history. You don't need to re-traumatize yourself every time a new resident comes to your child's hospital room. The same thing goes for relatives or friends—sharing the scary stuff can be a huge support, but no one is entitled to your stories. Save your energy and empathy for the people who actually need it—your child, their siblings, and your partner.

On Not Knowing

For all the reasons above, I think that knowing the cause of your child's deafness is a positive thing. It's not always a realistic thing, though. In the old days (like when *Frasier* was still on the air), it was common for parents not to know why their babies were deaf, and there are still plenty of cases of *idiopathic* deafness out there.

> When my first daughter was born, she was referred on her newborn hearing screen. It took 12 months for her to receive her identification of a mild bilateral hearing levels. The ENT mentioned that genetics and an MRI were natural next steps if we wanted more information about her, but our military insurance wasn't the greatest so we opted not to find out.
>
> A few months later I was pregnant with her sister. She was also identified with a mild hearing level at 1 month. We opted to speak with the genetic counselor, but testing was going to be well over $1500 out of pocket. This was not a cost our family could assume at the time.
>
> Two years later, and under different insurance, our third child was born. She also had a bilateral mild hearing level. We met with genetics again, and they offered a new test—this one was covered. We waited weeks for the test to come back, and when it did, it found no genetic markers for having a hearing difference. The geneticist was flabbergasted; he recommended coming back in 10 years when technology has time to catch up.
>
> Now, with the completion of our family, we are 4 for 4 deaf. Because our kids are healthy and there are no significant other syndromic health issues, we are at peace. Not knowing the origins of our children's hearing difference is a mystery, but accepted. For us, genetic information would not have changed our family size goals, it would not change the educational opportunities or what hearing aids the audiologist would offer. It would just be information.

Research suggests that there are higher levels of psychological well-being in Deaf adults who understand why or how they became Deaf, so in another 5 years or so, we may choose to seek testing again. When we do, our children will also be old enough to weigh in on those decisions as well.

Joanna, hearing parent and activist

The Autism Spectrum

Unlike pediatric deafness, which is relatively rare, "autism spectrum disorder (ASD)"[32] is one of the most common diagnoses for children. The CDC estimates that one in every thirty-six kids is on the spectrum. There is evidence that deafness and autism may be linked in some cases, but the raw math means that, whatever the reason, there are a lot of deaf autistic kids out there, with a huge range of needs and abilities.

If you have a deaf autistic child, finding the right therapeutic and educational environment for them can be tricky. Your local early intervention may struggle to get appropriate services to your kid, and the average program for autistic children is not set up for deaf kids. Unfortunately, the average deaf school may not have strong support for them, either—services for neurodivergent kids vary widely in deaf schools, and programs that might be great for neurotypical kids can have serious gaps or deficiencies for deaf autistic students, or just not the right balance of services for *your* child in particular. There are deaf schools with strong support or even dedicated programs to serve deaf autistic kids, but you may have to look across state lines to find the right fit.

Autism being so common, it can also be the first guess when your child begins to exhibit behavioral issues and language delays. Neurotypical deaf kids on the down-low can look an awful lot like hearing autistic kids because of similar communication frustrations, affect differences, and other issues. Getting a solid diagnosis when there may be an autism / deaf overlap is going to be tricky and will require deaf-savvy assessors who know and can unpick the various manifestations of both. Also, keep in mind that even if they have

---

[32]Like hearing loss, many advocates object to the term autism spectrum disorder because of its negative and inaccurate connotations, but it is still commonly used in medical settings. I'm avoiding it in this book where I can.

typical hearing, speech and / or auditory processing is sometimes a challenge for neurodivergent kids, and they may have better access to communication in Deaf environments where ASL is used.

The adult Deaf and Autism communities have many parallels; these are groups that were often subject to misguided and sometimes abusive interventions as children, along with misunderstandings and bigotry about their capacity as adults. They have common ground in activism, with many of the same interests around access to education and employment, fighting ableism and linguicism (discrimination based on language), and the recognition that their identities are not illnesses but are an expression of essential human diversity. They also find themselves in conflict with advocacy organizations headed primarily by parents or professionals. Looking for the experts on autism means looking for those autistic adults who can bring their own experiences to the table alongside their understanding of current research and best practices. To start, contact groups headed by autistic leaders like the Autistic Self Advocacy Network or their state affiliates.

Glue Ear and Ear Tubes / Grommets

AKA the dreaded *otitis media with effusion*, glue ear is a super-common childhood ailment where extra fluid gets trapped behind the eardrum in the middle ear. One in five children gets it at some point, often due to an ear infection, and generally it's NBD—it frequently resolves without treatment. Kids with conductive or mixed-type deafness are more likely to experience glue ear as a chronic issue, though, as they're more likely to have anatomical troubles with their *eustachian tubes*. These are the channels that connect the middle ear to the back of your throat and allow it to drain naturally. Long-term or recurrent glue ear might damage your kid's residual hearing, so if your child is prone to ear infections or has had glue ear in the past, it's important to talk with your doctor and audiologist about recognizing signs that it may return.

There are a variety of treatments if your child has glue ear, like the Valsalva maneuver (pinch your nose and blow out), a funky nose balloon, or medication like antibiotics or antihistamines. The most involved is a common surgical procedure called myringotomy or tympanostomy, which involves cutting a small vent in the eardrum to let the fluid out. Besides reducing infections, pain, and helping with balance issues caused by lingering goo, this can help deaf kids hear more by equalizing the pressure between the middle and outer ear and allowing the eardrum to vibrate more freely.

Once the hole is cut, doctors will often want to hold it open using *tympanostomy tubes*. Also just called *ear tubes* or *grommets*, they create a channel through the eardrum to allow fluid to drain from the middle ear to the outer ear. Tubes are small and temporary; the eardrum slowly closes over them and spits them out, usually leaving no hole behind. They can be in place for anywhere from six months up to four years, depending on different factors. Surgery to install grommets is very common, and risks are generally low, but they do require sedation and sometimes a second surgery if they don't pop out or if the eardrum doesn't fully close afterward.

Tinnitus

The last medical issue I want to flag is tinnitus, a ringing or humming in the ears. It's another super-common condition for both deaf and hearing folks (I'm experiencing some mild tinnitus right now), but in some deaf people, especially adults, it can be a heavy burden and interfere with daily life. Kids are much less likely to notice or be bothered by tinnitus, but be aware that it's a possibility, and if your child seems restless, anxious, or distracted, it may be what's bugging them. For some kids, putting on their hearing devices helps with tinnitus, while others respond better to white noise or music, or even psychotherapy or meditation techniques to learn to tune out the buzz.

Hearing Devices Quick Start Guide

Like I said in the first chapter, there are a number of different technologies your kid might use to access sound. Because there's a wide array of devices and manufacturers, I'm only going to cover the basics. If you want particular information about different brands, you will want to ask your audiologist or go to the manufacturer's website.[33]

---

[33]While I'm pretty critical of the ways they market hearing devices, device makers will be able to give you the most accurate technical information, and audiologists should be able to explain it in the context

Also keep in mind that this isn't Baskin-Robbins and you don't have your pick of flavors. Which prosthetic (if any) is appropriate for your child depends on their diagnosis, anatomy, and preferences. Your audiologist will be able to give you information about your kid's specific options, and you can go from there.

Babies versus Technology

A critical thing to remember about hearing devices: hearing aids and cochlear implants are marvels of modern electronics, but they're ONLY electronics. Ultimately, you're sticking thousands of dollars' worth of plastic, metal, and silicon, that have to be adjusted and situated juuuust right onto or *into*, your baby's head and hoping for the best.

Think about your cell phone. If it were your only means of communication, how often would you be cut off from the world? Now give your cell phone to a barfing, pooping baby and make it small enough to swallow. BAHAs, HAs, and CIs have batteries that die, parts that fall off, ear molds that need refitting, tubes that get wet, and coils that won't hold. You can't (well, you *shouldn't*) wear them to bed or in the bath, and they get knocked off by car seats, stuck to the fridge, and chewed up by the family dog.

And this is not just the hardware—software can fail, too. When the only person who can tell is the baby, you can go weeks or months with malfunctioning devices and not know it. Last year, several Australian hospitals were found to have incorrectly programmed ("mapped") the CIs of hundreds of children, preventing them from getting useful input from their devices. Despite these problems starting as early as 2008, they were only identified in 2023. Some kids suffered through decades of surgery, exams, and speech therapy, enduring terrible language deprivation, and *no professional noticed.*

This is another reason why having sign language in your pocket is a good idea—it can be *stressful* to manage devices. My kid has dropped his CIs into gutters, abandoned them in sandboxes, and recently anointed his brand new

---

of your child's particular situation. Just keep in mind that as soon as they start talking about things like education and language acquisition, they'll be speaking from the far end of the tube.

left-side Cochlear America Nucleus N8 processor in the crystal waters of Yosemite Falls. It never ends. While I always keep a sharp eye on his doodads, knowing ASL means we're never stuck for communication.

Hearing Aids (HAs)

The classic and most common hearing prosthetic. Recent regulatory and market changes (those Costco HAs) mean that they're everywhere these days—you might be using one right now. Essentially, hearing aids make things louder; they take in sound via a microphone, boost and filter the signal to make it more comprehensible, and then play it back into the ear canal using a tiny speaker.

Because of the level of amplification deaf kids often need, and because their ear canals grow fast, their hearing aids are usually the more powerful over-the-ear type, rather than the little chickpea things that fit entirely in your ear hole. Over-the-ear HAs generally use a mic sitting just above the ear and pipe audio into the ear through a tube attached to an ear mold, which is a tight-fitting, custom-cast silicone plug that needs to be continuously redone as your baby's ear canals get bigger. Loose-fitting molds cause squealy feedback and sore ears, so you'll be friends with your audiologist before long.

HAs take advantage of whatever residual hearing your kid has and can be tuned to amplify specific frequencies, filter, pitch-shift, or otherwise process sound to make it more accessible to them. Ultimately, though, a hearing aid can only do a certain amount; it can't add detail or unscramble speech so it's more intelligible, and your child has to have some level of hearing to begin with. For my son, who has zero residual hearing, HAs did nothing—we might as well have stuck gum in there.

Bone-Anchored Hearing Aids (BAHAs)

BAHAs are another very common tool for kids with conductive deafness, but one you may not know about. BAHAs are similar to conventional hearing aids; they take advantage of your child's residual hearing, but instead of making sounds louder and blasting them into the ear canal, they conduct those vibrations into your kid's skull; it's pretty badass. This works for children whose anatomy stops sound somewhere in the outer or middle ear, opening up an alternate channel of transmission for vibes to reach the inner ear and cochlea. If you've ever touched a tuning fork to your head and heard the note, it's the same concept. There are actually some fancy bone conduction headphones that use this method instead of conventional speakers.

For a BAHA to function, it needs to be pressed firmly against the head, so kids generally start with *softbands*, which are removable sweatband-like holders that keep them in place. When they are old enough, they can get a metal post or magnetic plate attached under their skin behind the ear. This gives the BAHA a sturdy anchor point to the skull and better sound conduction. These plates are generally installed in twos, so that if one is damaged, it's simple to set up the next one without more elaborate surgery. Although the initial surgery isn't too invasive, these sites can get infected or have other medical complications. And kids whose cochleas or auditory nerves don't transmit sound for whatever reason won't get any benefit from them.

CROS and BiCROS Systems

Sometimes just called *cross systems,* these are devices for kids with either single-sided deafness or different residual hearing levels in each ear. CROS systems look like a pair of hearing aids, but they capture sound from the deaf ear and route it to the hearing ear, giving your child 360° access to sound. BiCROS systems do the same thing but also boost the volume and process the sound like a conventional hearing aid.

These systems are sometimes overlooked because unilateral kids "still have one good ear," or ignored in favor of getting a CI in the deaf ear, but mixing down the stereo into a single channel can work very well in situations like school or sports where sound and voices are coming from all directions, and can give kids with SSD a boost to their auditory language exposure and comprehension without CI surgery.

Cochlear Implants (CIs)

The bionic option. CIs come in two parts: the processor and the implant. The processor stays outside your child's body, and it looks pretty much like a hearing aid or BAHA, although it works completely differently. Processors have microphones on them that gather sound, which is then gets doctored in various ways and translated into a magnetic pulse. This pulse is sent through your child's skin to a receiver on the implant, surgically placed under their scalp. The implant converts the magnetic signal into an electrical charge, which then travels to a string of electrodes curled into your child's cochlea, deep in their inner ear, zapping it in the appropriate places and creating a sound-like sensation.

CIs are different from hearing aids because they don't rely on residual hearing. They don't amplify anything and don't have speakers in them at all—that scene from *A Quiet Place* where they kill the monster with CI feedback was bullshit. This means that some kids, like my son, who had zero residual hearing but intact cochleas and functioning auditory nerves, can get cochlear implants and use them to access sound.

Middle Ear Implants (MEIs)

These are basically implantable hearing aids that work in various ways to address conductive deafness. They're not used in children under age five, so we'll leave them alone.

Auditory Brainstem Implants (ABIs)

Just no. These are systems that work similarly to CIs, but worse. Instead of the inner ear, an array of electrodes is implanted on the surface of the brain in the area that governs hearing, which communicates with an external processor. The processor passes magnetic signals to the implant, which translates them into electrical signals and zaps the brain to create a soundlike impression. This has the benefit of routing around missing or malfunctioning auditory nerves, but has the disadvantage of *parking something directly on the surface of your kid's brain.*

I'm trying to be even-handed in this section, but yikes. The outcomes for ABIs are generally worse than for CIs, and they are less likely to allow your child to understand spoken language. Hearing is optional, sign language exists, and brain surgery is just not worth it.

> *Eight Reasons You **Shouldn't** Learn Sign Language for Your kid*
> - Who cares what babies think?
> - You gotta trust nineteenth-century medicine
> - Let the scuba divers have their fun
> - Makes it too easy for the Patriots to steal your plays
> - It's not polite to openly gossip about strangers at the restaurant
> - Too many Oscar winners in your family already
> - Being a loudmouth chatterbox is kind of your *thing*
> - Because your kid's hearing technology works perfectly and never breaks

Cochlear Implant FAQ

CIs are possibly the most controversial medical technology this side of lip filler. This has a lot to do with their semi-permanent nature and the way that they are marketed as a "solution" to deafness, which they certainly are not.

Do CIs "Cure Deafness?" Do CIs Allow a Deaf Kid to Have "Normal Hearing?"

No. CIs are prosthetics that can give your child more access to sound. Kids with CIs are still deaf; when the processors come off, the sound goes with it. And even if implants work as intended, their experience of hearing is going to be different. It's kind of like making soup in a microwave versus a stovetop. You still get hot soup, but the steps in between aren't the same.

Typical human hearing has tens of thousands of channels, distinguishing between many pitches at once and giving a vast amount of detailed information. In comparison, CIs have a limited number of channels—it varies depending on the device and the way it interacts with your kid's body—but the total is somewhere between about twenty and a hundred-odd "virtual" channels, which are mediated by microphone technology, signal processing, and other factors. Adults who receive CIs after losing their hearing often report that the sensation is robotic, like the whole world was Autotuned. This is because CIs are boiling down a huge spectrum of sound into a relative handful of discrete tones.

In part because of these differences, listening to language via a CI can require a lot more attention, interpretation, and focus. For hearing people, sliding between passive reception and active listening is automatic. You can be grabbing a drink at a noisy party and tune out most of the audio clutter, but then snap to attention when you hear someone call your name and shift to a one-on-one conversation when your friend arrives with some juicy gossip. We tend to take those transitions in hearing and attention for granted, but for kids with CIs—and for kids using hearing technology of any kind—they can require an enormous and active effort. This is why deaf kids get listening fatigue—they're literally burning more calories per word just trying to understand speech.

Does Your Kid *Need* CIs?

No. Your kid needs *language*, spoken or signed. Some SLPs or audiologists will oversell CIs as being "language implants," but CIs are no more language implants than your thumbs are Mario Kart implants. They are one potential way to get your child language, but they're not the only, or even the most reliable way. Even if your child is a good candidate for them, cochlear implant surgery is purely elective. It's not abuse or neglect to not implant your deaf child, and no doctor on earth can force them on your baby without your consent. By the same token, though, it's not inherently wrong or abusive to *get* your kid a CI. The decision to implant is complicated—ethically, medically, and educationally—and anybody telling you otherwise ain't your friend.

What Are Some Reasons *Not* to Get a CI?

Since the most common negative experience parents have is feeling hustled or pressured into implanting their kids, let's start with some completely valid reasons you can choose not to give your child CIs:

Your baby is whole and perfect just as they are. That's the unvarnished truth, and it is enough.

You don't want to subject your child to surgery or possible complications. CI implantation is not *brain* surgery, but it is *head* surgery that comes close to the braincase, and it does involve a certain amount of drilling into the skull. There will be vaccinations, hospitalization, sedation, sutures, healing, and rehabilitation. Complications with CIs are unusual, but complications involving your kid's head and ear anatomy can be serious; you definitely don't want to be dealing with infections, long-term pain, or involuntary nerve stimulation from the implant. And you might not want to subject your child to multiple surgeries if something goes wrong the first time. Kids tend to be rubbery and recover fast, but you're totally within your rights to skip it altogether.

Your kid is a marginal candidate and you feel like it's not worth the risk. Some children's anatomy or other medical issues mean that implants have a lower chance of working, or may carry more than the normal risk of complications. Sometimes surgeons are willing to roll the dice when the odds are bad—hearing professionals have an unfortunate tendency to focus on the best possible outcomes, rather than the most likely outcomes. But you get to look at the numbers, too, and decide to spare your kid the surgery and rehab if it's less likely to pan out.

You want to wait until your child is older so they can participate in the decision. CIs are a permanent change to a child's body and can have long-term side effects and maintenance costs. You might not be comfortable making that kind of decision for them or without their input. Whether that means waiting until they're a little older and you can have conversations about it, or waiting until they're young adults who can make the decision all on their own, this is a valid perspective.

You don't want to damage your child's residual hearing. The process of inserting an electrode into the cochlea interferes with the typical functioning of the inner ear and can disrupt whatever existing hearing your kid has. Although the technology and surgical techniques to preserve residual hearing are getting better, and some kids can retain hearing "around" the implant, you can decide it's not worth the risk or the trade-off.

You don't think it offers your kid a greater benefit than other hearing devices or no devices at all. The important thing is that they truly acquire a fluent first language early on, which is why sign is so critical. But for their "hearing needs," hearing aids, BAHAs, or CROS systems might be sufficient. It's really all about what works for *them*.

You don't want to saddle your child with the future difficulty and expense of maintaining it. CI implants last around thirty years before they need to be replaced, which will require another round of surgery. They need regular maintenance and updates in the meantime, and a good insurance policy to cover them.

There are no generic CI parts: external processors only work with implants from the same manufacturer, and while they work hard to make backward-compatible devices, your child may eventually find themselves with obsolete hardware in their head. The same goes for all consumable parts—coils, (some) batteries, mic covers, ear hooks, and so on. They wear out regularly and can only be bought from the manufacturer. So unlike hearing aids, once you have an implant by a certain maker, you're pretty much locked into their products for life, or at least the life of the implant. Being a cyborg is a lot, and it's reasonable not to want to impose that on your kid.

You don't want to give in to the pressure of doctors or family. People, both so-called professionals and the amateurs we call our loved ones, sometimes get really pushy or creepy about CIs. As the parent, if you're not convinced that they're the best option for your kid, it's your call.

You don't care if your baby can hear or not. Really just restating that first reason. Language is mandatory. Hearing is optional.

What Are Some *Good* Reasons to Get Your Kid a CI?

Ok, so if those are all reasons to say no, are there reasons to say yes? A lot of this book was written to help you think this through realistically, with perspectives from Deaf adults who have been there, but considering I got my kid a CI, yeah, I do think there are some good reasons:

It gives some kids better options for developing spoken language skills. For all that it's a different experience than "natural" hearing, mediated by a prosthetic, and not a reliable way to get an L1 into your child. CIs really do make pursuing spoken language possible for some kids who'd otherwise not have a realistic shot at it. Depending on their particular situation, if you want to give your child access to spoken English, CIs may be your best bet.

For receptive spoken language, earlier is better. The earlier your child has access to spoken language, the more likely they are to develop strong comprehension and speech skills themselves. The trade-off for waiting until your child is older and can participate in the decision to get a CI is that your child is less likely to have a big benefit from it. So, if your child was born with low levels of residual hearing, and you want them to develop strong spoken language skills, you will want to consider implanting them sooner rather than later. This isn't necessarily the situation with kids with higher levels of hearing or with progressive hearing loss—like everything else, it's a case-by-case consideration.

It gives your child access to a greater slice of the social/educational pie. I'm a huge fan of Deaf culture and Deaf education, and the evidence shows that kids with CIs have a better chance of thriving with ASL and Deaf culture than without. And kids who *don't* use hearing technology can absolutely be happy and successful without devices. But CIs can also give a child a chance for experiences they wouldn't otherwise be able to easily access. It's up to you to decide if it's worth the trade-offs and have options in place if the technology doesn't work out.

We do all sorts of things to our children that can't be undone. Although CIs are a permanent change to their body that will have long-term impacts on their life, this is only one of many similar decisions you as a parent will make for your child. After all, I cut the tip of my kid's penis off, too—I'm raising him Jewish, bilingual, a second sibling, with my values and with my cooking. These things will all mark him as permanently, if possibly less concretely, as having a CI. The law recognizes my capacity as a parent to make these choices for my kid, but what's *legal* is really the first and lowest hurdle when you're thinking about what's *right*.

Bad Reasons

Bad reasons to get CIs can look a lot like good reasons; like the kids say, you've got to interrogate your motives. But bad reasons can poison your relationship with your child, putting enormous and unreasonable pressure on them to work with an all-too-fallible technology, be "normal," and to be like you. Our children, deaf and hearing, will always be different from us. With a deaf kid, you just learn that a little sooner.

I want to fix my child's deafness. Your child is not broken. You *cannot* go into this process with that perspective. Believing this *will* break your child, and it can break you and your family into a million pieces along the way.

CIs are the easiest option. Don't get your child a CI to make it "easier"—for you or your family. Whatever else is going on in your life, you're the grown-up—you have the ability to make decisions and do hard work like learning ASL.[34] Your baby can't make those choices, and by relying on the CIs alone, you're expecting a child to put in all the effort and take all the risks. Like my wife says, don't meet your kid halfway, meet them all the way. The burden is on you.

I want my kid to fit into their family or the hearing world. I hate to be the bearer of bad news, but your child is deaf; fitting into the hearing world is not necessarily an easy or realistic goal, whether or not they have CIs, and forcing the issue is one of the key sources of misery for many deaf folks growing up. No one wants our children to struggle more than they need to, but CIs don't magically make life simpler for them—and they sometimes add to the challenges. Ultimately, your child is the one who decides where and how they fit into the rest of your family. Accepting that they are deaf is more important than whether you get them implants or not.

I want my child to hear the birds, aka "I couldn't live without music." It's hard to imagine our own lives without the things we cherish, and it's natural to want to share what we love with our kids. But our children's lives are their own, and they will find their joy. Plenty of deaf people enjoy music with or without CIs, of course, but if your kid doesn't "do" music? What about dance or cooking barbecue? Playing hockey, playing video games, making art, or doing BMX racing? There are whole worlds out there that don't need sound. It does you no good and can do your kid a great deal of harm to lay your expectations on them.

I am also sad to report that, whether you love Bach, Beyoncé, or REO Speedwagon, if your deaf child does have access to music, they will instantly gravitate toward whatever you find grating and inane. That's just how it works.

---

[34]LSL and other not-good forms of speech therapy can be an enormous of work for parents, but it's still starting from a place of familiarity and comfort: English.

CIs Now and Later

A critical part of making the CI decision for your kid is looking at the long-term outcomes for kids with CIs. When you ask doctors about this, you'll often get information about the *failure rate* of CIs for children, which hovers between three and seven percent.[35]

These are good numbers to know, but they only tell a small part of the story. "Failure" in this case means device failure: either the actual physical doohickey breaks, a *hard failure*, or it fails to give comprehensible or tolerable input, a *soft failure*, or there's a secondary medical complication like an infection that forces the implant to get taken out.

For one thing, this does mean that about one in twenty kids who get CIs will need to have them removed or reimplanted; no matter what the odds are on paper, it sucks to be that kid. For another, that number doesn't cover the periodic device recalls CI companies have had to announce, where *all* models of possibly flawed or defective implants need to get pulled and replaced for children's safety.[36]

Most importantly, this failure rate doesn't say anything about actually being able to understand and use spoken language. There's a spectrum of language outcomes that kids with CIs have, and "device not broken" is just the start. For a CI (or any other hearing technology) to be useful for your child, it has to meet three different sets of standards:

Medical-Audiological

Does your child's anatomy permit them to use a CI? Is the implant intact? Does it deliver sound?

This is where the three-to-seven percent reported failure rate comes in. Kids like to dive headfirst off high places, so they have the highest rate of hard

---

[35] Manufacturers reported lower rates of failure, while hospitals and surgeons tended to report higher rates.

[36] Every CI company has had to recall implanted parts, most recently Advanced Bionics in 2020, which recalled all its HiRes Ultra and Ultra 30 implants.

failures, but, depending on whose research you look at, soft failures are almost as common. Thankfully, medical complications seem to be much more rare in children, but they certainly do happen.

Doctors and hospitals that do a lot of CI surgeries tend to have lower rates of failure and complications, and if you are considering a CI, you should be asking for the ENT's statistics to be certain you're getting someone who's experienced. This is also an area where you should be very aggressive about identifying your child's risk factors: among other reasons, if they have atypical cochleas or auditory nerves, or if they became deaf due to meningitis, this can raise the risk of the CI not working, and you should factor it into the cost / benefit analysis.

Linguistic

Can your kid take the beeps and bloops that the implant delivers to them and interpret that sound into *language*? Can they use that input as a basis to build strong receptive and expressive oral language skills?

This is where the rubber meets the road; kids can sit in the audiologist's booth all day, raising their hands when they hear a tone, and still struggle to sort those frequencies out into comprehensible speech in the real world. **About seventy percent of school-age children with CIs don't have age-appropriate language abilities.**[37]

To take the medical model seriously for a moment, if CIs really were a pill to cure language deprivation, and they only worked thirty percent of the time, it might not be the first pill you'd reach for. The metaphor isn't really fair, though, because it's not that CIs are bad at teaching kids English—it's that CIs can't teach kids anything. They're not language teaching machines; implants can create a *channel* to access sound, but one that's not fully open for many children.

---

[37] It's important to note that most of those kids are in mainstream / monolingual programs with little to no ASL. If you look at kids who *have* early access to ASL, whether they have CIs or not, they tend to have more typical language skills.

Educational-Social-Functional

What's it like to use the CI day in and day out? Does the implant give your child headaches or have other obnoxious side effects? How hard is it to learn using an implant in school? How nice is it to play with friends or watch a movie while using CIs? This is the last hurdle devices need to clear: do they make your child's life any better, from *their* point of view?

About forty percent of kids who get implants as children stop using them by the time they're eighteen. CIs never really worked for some of these kids. For others, it's just too tiring, annoying, or painful, even if they can use them to understand spoken language. Others may have found other ways of getting access that work better for them.

When I look at how Deaf adults use their hearing devices, it seems a little like riding a bicycle. Not only do you need to know how to ride a bike and have a bike available, but you also need a *reason* to ride it. You might love your bike and take it every day to work. Or you might only ride your bike on weekends for fun. You might hate riding your bike and only do it when your car is in the shop, or you might just ditch your bike and get some sweet rollerblades.

These are all things adult CI (and HA) users do, too—some rely on their technology for most of their daily communication, some use it just for stuff like music or movies, and some only use it when they absolutely have to, or not at all. Where your kid eventually falls on that spectrum doesn't determine if the CI was "worth it" or not; ultimately that's something only your kid can decide for themselves. Just don't put all your eggs in one basket, is what I'm saying.

Hearing Aid, CROS, and BAHA FAQ

Now that we've definitively answered every medical, ethical, and educational question about CIs, let's talk more generally about hearing technology.

Does My Kid Need a Hearing Device?

No, your kid needs language. Just as with CIs, other hearing-related doodads are a potential channel to learn language through, but they aren't magic

English-teaching devices. Kids with low levels of residual hearing may or may not get much benefit from them in terms of understanding speech.[38] It's very much individual, and you'll need to experiment and see what works for them. If your child doesn't get good access to spoken English via HAs or BAHAs, and they are well-supported with ASL, you might end up skipping technology altogether.

On the other hand, for kids with mild or moderate deafness, or who are deaf in only one ear, hearing technology can be a big help, especially if their education is more focused on spoken language. Sometimes parents or misguided professionals will want these kids to tough it out and get by just with whatever hearing they have, with the idea that they won't become "dependent" on devices. But research shows that children in the mild-moderate range, or who are unilaterally deaf, really benefit from the extra information they get from hearing technology and have better language outcomes because of it.

Does My Kid Need to Wear Their Technology All Day?

No. Some audiologists and SLPs will insist on an "eyes open, ears on" policy, but for young children it's not helpful or realistic to expect them to wear hearing aids, CROS systems, BAHAs, or CIs all waking hours. When your kid first gets their devices, you might only get a few minutes of on-time daily. That will hopefully increase as your baby gets used to the feeling of having the gadget attached to their body, along with the added sensory stimulation. Oscar was a sensory freak and LOVED his CIs as a baby, but even he would burn out eventually—the veins would pop out of his neck and he'd start blowing up other people's heads, *Scanners* style.

As time goes on, your child may start to appreciate the extra sound information they're getting—they can hear their own screams!—and get into a positive feedback loop of wanting to wear their devices so they can hear more stuff, which gives them more time and practice with the devices, making it easier to wear them for longer. On the other hand, your child might not like

---

[38] There are reasons to use hearing technology other than just language acquisition and perception, including access to music, environmental sound awareness, and management of tinnitus.

the sensations that hearing technology gives them. You can then end up in a negative feedback loop where they dislike their devices, and so you struggle to get them to wear them, and so they learn to hate it when you try to make them wear the things they hate, and so on.

Keep in mind that all kids, whether they enjoy their devices or not, get listening fatigue and will do better with periodic breaks. Working your way into a routine helps to make wearing devices a little easier, but if your baby is struggling with their hearing device, you can always take a break and put the aids away for an hour, a day, or a week, however long you need that cool-off period. In the meantime, you can keep communicating and building their language and cognitive skills with ASL. If the device stays in the drawer, that's fine.

Oscar got CIs activated at about eight months, and by the time he was a year old, he was averaging four to five hours of wear time daily, which was enough for him to build a strong basis in spoken English along with ASL. Now that he's older, he wears his CIs for maybe eight hours a day. He likes to put them in the car on the way to school, to talk with me and listen to the Bluey soundtrack, and then he leaves them on most of the day at his deaf school—where he absolutely doesn't need them. After school, he'll probably spend about half the evening with them on, especially if he's due for some TV, but he has this weird thing where he takes them (and all the rest of his clothes) off to poop, and he tends to leave them off after that.

It can sometimes be frustrating to have a kid whose devices aren't reliably there—I've delivered more than one monologue before noticing that he's gone sound-off. But I'm very happy with the way he uses his CI, because it's all about what he wants and needs. We can sign, or we can talk. The only time we really fight about them is when he ditches them under the couch.

What's That Squeaking Noise, and How Do I Stop It?

Hearing aids are like any other sound system: if noise from the speaker makes its way back to the microphone, it will begin echoing back and forth in a hellish high-pitched shriek of feedback. This bothers some deaf kids, and it bothers *every* hearing parent.

Ear molds are part of the solution; by completely plugging the ear canal, they keep the sound moving in just one direction. The problems come when the molds aren't fitting tightly—either because they got jostled or because their ear holes have grown. In the first case, the easy fix is to stuff the molds back in and possibly hold them in place with a pilot cap or headband. In the second case, you will need to go back to the audiologist to get new molds made. Babies grow at a ferocious rate, including their ear canals, so a one-year-old might need new molds almost every month. It gradually slows down from there, but you will definitely be on a first-name basis with your audiologist by the time your kid hits kindergarten.

But besides poorly fitting molds, feedback is also caused by the mic pressing against things like headrests and mattresses. This is a problem for babies who can't hold their heads up, but be aware that it can also happen with hats and even your face—going in for a hug and kiss can create a painful squeal for your kid, so be careful.

Fucking Magnets, How Do They Work?

Hearing devices of all kinds are designed for the lumbering beasts called adults, not the wiggly little goo balls that are our babies. Wearing a hearing aid or CI processor loosely, relying on gravity to keep it on the ear, or a magnet to keep it stuck to the scalp, is basically impossible. Manufacturers have developed some accessories to help, but homegrown and Etsy-powered solutions are nearly as common and sometimes more effective:

Pilot or aviator caps (HA or CI): Goes over the ears and straps on the chin to prevent your child from touching their devices at all. I go back and forth on them—they're sort of hilarious and can be adorable, but they're also faintly medical and can seem a little punitive.

Headbands (HA, CI): I find most of the CI manufacturer's headbands unutterably ugly and medical-seeming, but some third-party bands have a cute 1980s athleisure or 1920s flapper vibe to them.

Softbands (BAHA): These need a tight fit to keep the device pressed against the skull for good sound conduction, and generally look like sock garters.

Ear molds (HA, CI): Not just for HAs, CIs can also be held in place with a "blank" ear mold that's just there for ergonomics.

Ear loops (CI): You can get silicone loops that anchor the device around the ear like rubber bands; it's worth a shot.

Wig Tape (CI, HA): The kind your audiologist typically gives out is not much better than a post-it note. RuPaul-strength wig tape is available from the beauty supply store.

Hats (CI): You can buy custom beanies and baseball caps with slots for CIs, but my wife and I came up with a homegrown solution that worked very well. You can check out the no-sew instructions at willfertman.com/bearhat.

How the Hell Am I Going to Pay for All This?

Hearing technology is really spendy. Generally, insurance companies and Medicaid are willing to cover cochlear implants and BAHAs, and given that the costs can run into the tens or hundreds of thousands of dollars for surgery plus devices, almost nobody would have them if they didn't.

Hearing aids and CROS systems are often not paid for by insurance (although Medicaid families usually have coverage). Their price tag is generally lower than CIs and BAHAs, but they can still run several thousand dollars per device. Some states have mandates that require insurance to cover hearing aids or have public hearing aid support for low-income families, but it varies state to state and plan to plan—here in California, as of 2024, the hearing aid program is very difficult to qualify for, and it's tough to find audiologists who participate. Your local deaf services agency is a good place to start looking for information on this topic.

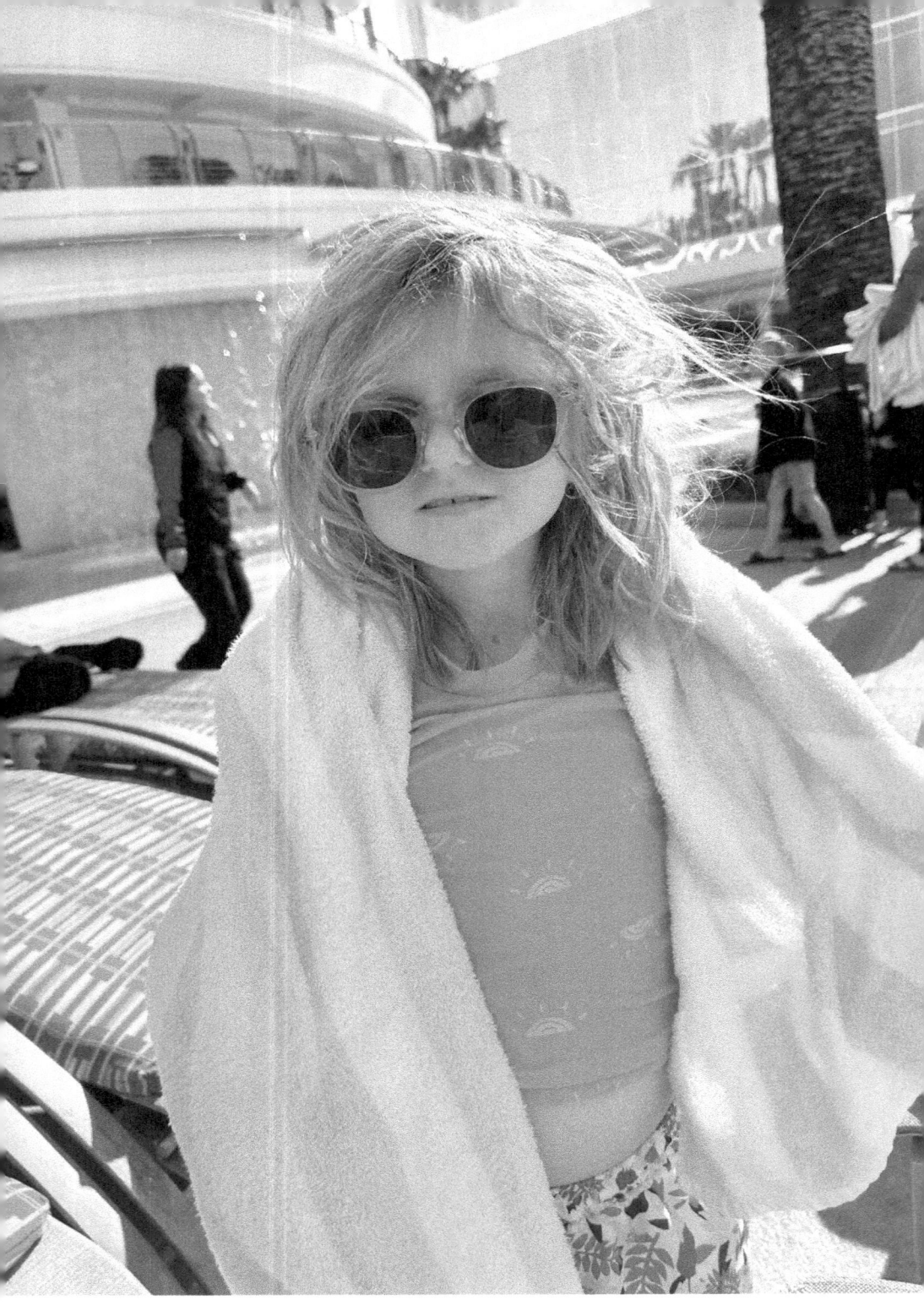

Sam Graydon, 2025

5

Dealing with It

I get to flip tables only once, in each part of my life. One time at work, one time for Oscar, and so on. After that, I have to deal with my shit, so I don't become "that woman who flips tables."

my wife

Anger

Somewhere in this process you will become angry. You're going to be mad at yourself, your partner, your family, your kids. You'll get mad at teachers, strangers, genes, viruses, God, and the phone company. Moms in particular can experience a lot of pressure to "not be angry" about some really spectacular bullshit. Dads sometimes get the opposite treatment: deference to anger that's designed to smooth it over without actually solving problems, leaving you ready for another bout of useless rage.

People like to talk about anger as a motivator, as the energy you use to change the world. But the world is big; just pouring your rage into it raw is like pissing in the reservoir. *You* might feel some relief, but plenty of fish got there before you did, and you're only setting yourself up for a misdemeanor court appearance.

Although my family is past some of the scariest "deaf kid" bottlenecks, I struggle with anger every day; the impulse to murder the entire district administration never quite goes away. But a killing spree is probably not going to help me make it through drop-off tomorrow, let alone the next IEP meeting, and it's no secret that sitting on my anger will end up hurting the people I most want to protect.

Managing anger isn't one thing, it's a whole set of skills. You have got to be willing to walk away from a situation when you're going to blow up. You need to communicate with your partner so you can catch one another when you're falling. You need to build stress-free time into your week. You also need to start picking apart exactly *what* you're angry about. Like literally everything else in this book, you do not have time to do these things, but they're important. You'll need practice, and it definitely helps to have a therapist.

Using rage to make a difference means waiting—not holding it in forever, but learning how to acknowledge it and temper it with love, compassion, and patience. When you're furious, use that moment to set a real goal: get that therapy approved for your kid, or tell your sister she's not welcome for Christmas, or learn the next ten signs in the workbook. Then take a second to forgive yourself, do some deep breathing, then take the anger and piss it into a jar—don't throw it away, but get it out of you. Talk to someone who's on your side, and put it somewhere where you can return to it every once in a while, give it a shake, and understand it better. Let it mellow, and add some love to it, so when you finally take it down off the shelf, at the right moment, it'll have turned from piss into gasoline. Then you can start lighting some fires.

Snappy Answers to Stupid Questions

When you have a deaf kid, the inane questions come so thick and fast that it's helpful to have a few canned responses in your pocket, especially when you're stuck on a plane next to an amateur speech pathologist. So here are some useful phrases you can deploy to amuse yourself and shame friends, relatives, and strangers in lieu of strangling them. Deaf people get these *a lot*, so if you're reading this, I apologize if I ripped yours off and didn't give proper credit.

Does your kid lip-read?

- Why, do you lipwrite?
- No, but she can handtalk.
- If the gossip's really good.
- Well, technically the full process is called speechreading, and it's really more of a supplemental receptive language skill that some deaf individuals use in combination with residual hearing because as you know only approximately 30 percent of English phonemes are visible

on the exterior of the mouth; the remainder of which are generally produced internally by the tongue, palate, larynx, and pharynx working in concert. This typically leaves a great deal of additional information to be inferred by context, which isn't developmentally appropriate for a toddler's L1, so instead we chose to pursue a natural signed language.
- Yes, and she told me what *you* said.

How will they make friends?

- Paper-maché and pipe cleaners.
- Gift certificates and a generous return policy.
- A sparkling personality and unlimited Labubu budget.
- The same way you did, by asking such *thoughtful* questions!
- My kid won't make friends, they will only *steal* friends from other kids.

Have you heard about this amazing new technology called cochlear implants?

- His cochleas are big enough, thanks.
- I'm not into gardening.
- No, I only have a two-year-old deaf child. Nobody ever told me about those!
- Yes, I found out about them through this amazing new technology called the World Wide Web!
- We're waiting until she's old enough to watch *Terminator* before going full cyborg.

My dog is deaf!

- And colorblind!
- Have you heard about this amazing new technology called cochlear implants?
- How will they learn to drive?
- Wow! Who's your dog's audiologist?
- How does she hear Timmy when he's fallen down the well?

I'm so sorry your child is deaf!

- That was YOU?[1]
- But that National Park Access pass is such a great deal!
- We were aiming for blind. Can't win 'em all, I guess.
- To think of all the wonderful people like you that he'll never get a chance to really know.
- Not me. I'm ready to become a deaf kid stage dad. Look out, Nyle DiMarco!

---

[1]Thanks to Bee Vickars for this one.

I'm so sorry your child is dead!

- Autocorrect much?

But how will they drive?

- Like this: <make car noises> <pretend to drive> <run away>
- Ever see *Baby Driver*?
- They'll just use a Deaf car.
- Just like daredevil stuntwoman and professional racer Kitty O'Neil.
- So you're like, the last person on earth to get a Deaf Uber?

Aren't you worried about them getting a job?

- So you're like, the last person on earth to get a Deaf Uber?
- I know! Those White House internships are SO competitive!
- Two words: underwater welding.
- I mean, have you seen *your* kid? Let's not throw stones here.
- He'll be ok. We're teaching him to photosynthesize.

If he can hear with his hearing aids, why are you sending him to the deaf school?

- Your kid can walk with their walking legs. Why are you sending them to sitting school?
- *Deaf* school? I thought it was *Death* school. Guess I need my hearing checked too!
- It's my best shot at deaf grandkids.
- Have you been to the cafeteria? The nuggets are *to die for!*
- The owl just kept delivering invitations.

What does it feel like to be deaf?

- What does it smell like to be you?

Would you like the braille menu?[2]

- We would prefer the scratch 'n sniff menu.

I will pray for your child

- But will you *tithe* for my child?
- Careful! The Devil knows sign language too![3]
- Oh good, I'll send you the Amazon Wishlist.
- It only counts if it's in ASL.
- Is your God Deaf too?

---

[2]Sighted Deaf adults get asked this—seriously.

[3]Thanks to Carrie for this one.

> **You are on an amazing journey**
> - Thanks! The grocery store *is* pretty great.
> - Namaste. <give them the finger>
> - More like an amazing *joyride*. <steal their car>
> - So are you! <push them down the stairs>
> - Yes, but I'd still like my frappuccino, thanks.

Last Story Before Bed

There is nothing harder than being a parent. Your heart escapes your chest and stumbles around on its own, bumping into sharp corners and putting things in its mouth. And when you're raising a deaf child, it can feel like there's darkness on every side. Some days it's unrelenting—on top of the daily grind of diapers, feedings, early wake-ups, and botched nap times, there can be medical crises, language struggles, dipshit administrators sabotaging your kid's IEP, or budget cuts that run straight through the one good program in your state.

But the way forward isn't a mystery. The Deaf community is there, ready for your child and your family. And there are good professionals, Deaf and hearing, who can guide you, even from hundreds of miles away. There are soft landings, too—nobody is a perfect parent, and our kids bounce back from our mistakes a lot faster than we do.

There is nothing better than being a parent. Sometimes, joy will tear through you like lightning, and the flash will light up the darkness. You'll see far ahead, to a place where your child is grown, happy, and walking their own road. And if you're prepared for the shock, and you're ready to catch it, you can conduct that charge through your body and share its glow and its warmth with your baby.

They'll never see the smoke.

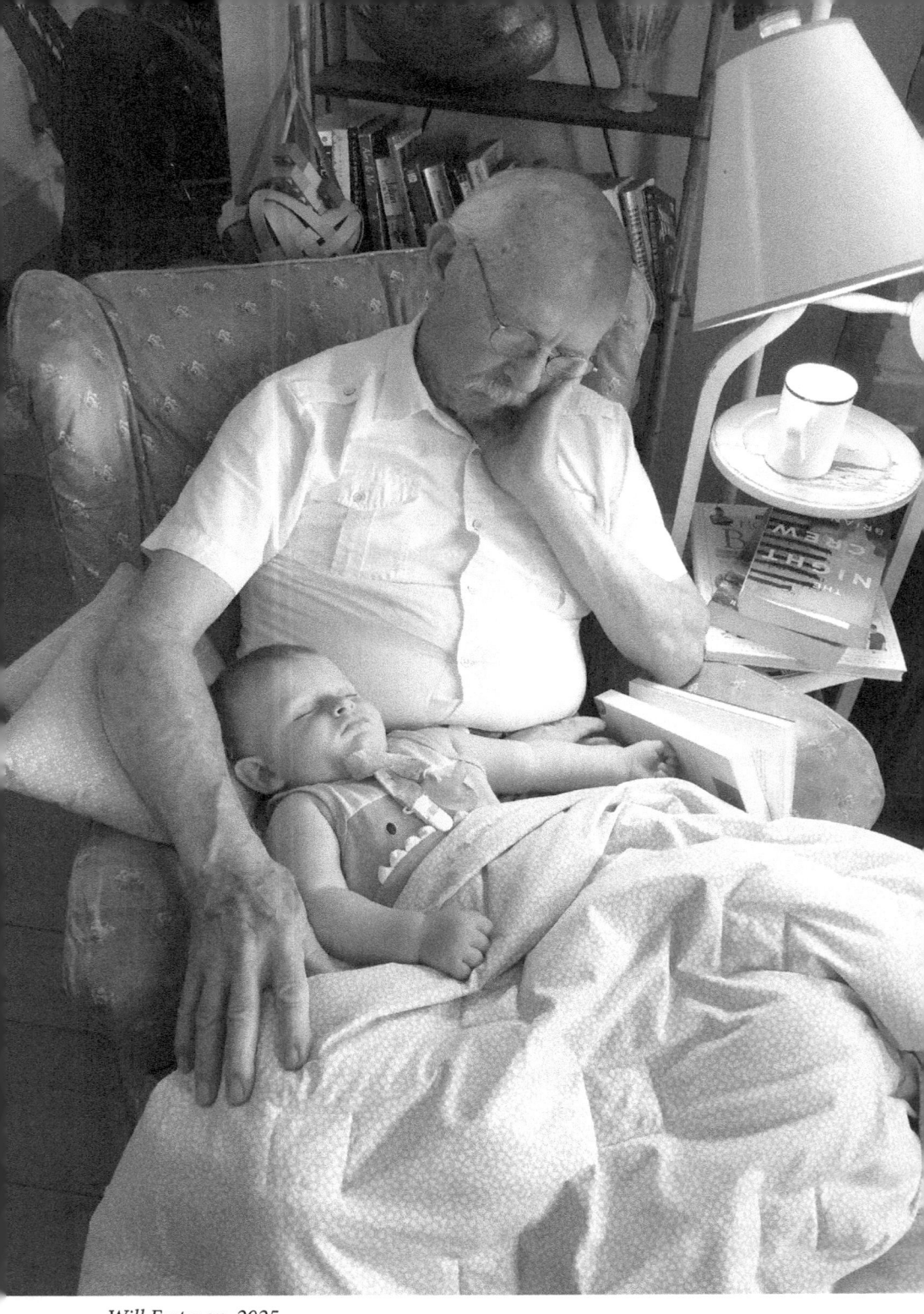
Will Fertman, 2025

Glossary

Social Terms

There is some specialized vocabulary used by and about Deaf people, their communities, and experiences that you should know:

Audism: Discrimination based on hearing status. Deaf author Tom Humphries defined the term in 1977 as *"The notion that one is superior based on one's ability to hear or behave in the manner of one who hears."* You'll see this word a lot because there's a lot of it out there. It can be blatant, as when my kid's Deaf sitter was refused service at our local YMCA, or it can be subtle, as when a school administrator "forgets" to mention the local Deaf services agency in your IFSP onboarding.

> **linguicism:** Discrimination based on language, often but not always overlapping with audism. Comes up a lot because there's a lot of it out there. Like audism, linguicism can be blatant, when someone mocks child's speech, or subtle, as when a professional counts your child's English and not their ASL vocabulary in an assessment.

Children of Deaf Adults (CODA): Often used as an umbrella term for any hearing person with Deaf parents, it more specifically indicates adults over the age of eighteen. CODAs can be hearing or Deaf themselves, but the term typically indicates that the person has a connection to the big-D Deaf community. There are a couple of related terms:

> **Kids of Deaf Parents (KODA)**: Anyone under age of 18 with one or more Deaf parents is a KODA.

SODA, GODA and beyond: These are slangy backronyms and aren't universally recognized—SODA stands for Siblings of Deaf Adults or Kids, while GODA is Grandchild of Deaf Adults. Folks will sometimes invent new -ODAs purely for joke purposes: DODAs (Dogs of Deaf Adults,) LODAS (Lawyers of Deaf Adults,) PODeKs (Parents of Deaf Kids?!?) etc. Don't use these with a straight face.

Deaf, the Deaf community, "big-D Deaf": Folks without typical hearing who use ASL or another natural sign language and consider themselves part of a culturally and linguistically distinct group. This can be in addition to other identities—Black Deaf, Deaf Disabled, and so on; it's not an all-or-nothing thing.

Deaf culture: The culture and traditions people in the Deaf community share, starting with sign language and radiating out into other aspects of life. Includes practical things like habits around pointing or information-sharing, more abstract principles like mutual support, and artistic traditions like ASL storytelling. Deaf culture can also encompass non-deaf folks like CODAs who sign and who understand its values.

Deaf Bing: The quirks of Deaf people and Deaf culture: lightswitch flicking, Deaf Standard Time, frisbee golf, etc. "Bing" is from the mouthshape you make when signing TENDENCY.

deaf, "small-d deaf": Folks without typical hearing, whether they consider themselves culturally Deaf or not.

deaf and dumb: An offensive and outdated term for obvious reasons—besides "dumb" being a synonym for "stupid," it implies deaf people can't use their voice or can't communicate, neither of which is true. Do not use.

deaf mute: Also outdated and offensive for much the same reason. Also do not use.

See also *non-verbal* under *Medical and Audiological terms*

Deaf Disabled: Deaf people with additional disabilities. This covers everything from motor disabilities, intellectual disabilities, immunocompromised people, and so on. A very diverse community in itself.

Deaf Plus, Deaf +: Deaf people with additional disabilities. Sometimes used to refer specifically to Deaf people with intellectual or developmental disabilities, sometimes not.

DeafBlind: Folks who are both deaf and blind or have low vision and consider themselves part of a culturally and linguistically distinct group related to, but separate from, the Deaf community. DeafBlind folks sometimes use ProTactile, a sign language that uses touch as its modality.

deafblind: Deaf folks without typical vision, whether they consider themselves culturally DeafBlind or not.

hard of hearing (HoH or HH): A subjective label that people with many different hearing levels apply to themselves. It signals that a person has some level of hearing, either using technology or not, but does not indicate what forms of communication that person prefers or whether they consider themselves culturally Deaf or not.

Hearing loss: This one still gets used in the hearing world, but in the Deaf community, it's a borderline slur. The general objections are that it focuses on "loss" rather than anything positive, and for many Deaf folks, it's just not accurate—you can't lose what you never had. An exception is made when it actually describes someone's hearing levels decreasing—"progressive hearing loss."

> **hearing impaired:** also a borderline slur. Instead, use deaf or hard of hearing in conversation, depending on the situation.
>
> **Deaf Gain:** The advantages that being Deaf confer to a person, and which can be shared with hearing people as well; the opposite of "hearing loss." This can range from simple things like a good night's sleep or sharp peripheral vision to advances like the football huddle, closed captioning, or Beethoven's 9th symphony.

Late deafened: People like Ludwig van Beethoven who lose their hearing after early childhood. There's no official cutoff age, but it's generally applied to people who've already built significant language and social skills as hearing person, and for whom being deaf is a major adjustment.

Medical and Audiological Terms

What we talk about when we talk about "hearing loss." When at the doctor or audiologist's office, there is a set of common terms used to describe hearing levels and basic ear mechanics from a medical perspective. These terms get chained together to describe what's going on in a particular person. Because it's still common for medical professionals to use the term "hearing loss," rather than deaf or deafness, I've put both terms in here.

For instance, my kid is completely deaf in both ears from a neurological condition that affects his cochlea, so he's got (deep breath): *profound non-syndromic bilateral sensorineural deafness*. His friend was born with a small ear and narrow ear canal on just one side, so he has *moderate unilateral conductive deafness and microtia.*

Taken altogether, this system can create a kind of word salad where everyone has hyper-specific descriptions and nobody is like anyone else, but the Deaf community recognizes that there's a big difference between the various medical diagnoses of deafness, the highly personal experience of deafness, and the common social and cultural aspects of being deaf. This is why in Deaf spaces they typically leave these terms alone and stick with "Deaf."

Audiogram: A map of your child's hearing, showing at what volume and in which ear they can detect certain frequencies of sound.

    the speech banana: A smile-shaped area in the top-center of audiograms that defines the pitches associated with human speech. To hear people's voices, a kid must be able to hear frequencies that fall inside the speech banana, although that's not necessarily enough to understand spoken language.

    flat deafness / hearing loss: more or less the same level of deafness across all frequencies.

    sloping: a type of deafness where hearing levels drop as you move from higher to lower frequencies. Also called *ski-slope*, because that's where the audiologist is going for winter break.

    reverse slope: the opposite of sloping deafness—deafness in the high tones but greater hearing in the low tones. ::boom the bass::

cookie bite: deafness in the middle frequencies around human speech, but not high or low tones. Looks like a Muppet took a chomp out of the audiogram.
reverse cookie bite (!!!): hearing the middle frequencies but deafness in the high and low tones.

Auditory brainstem response (ABR) or auditory evoked potential (AEP) test: A very common hearing test given to newborns and infants. Electrodes are stuck to their head and sounds are played into their ears *while they sleep*. The electrodes measure brain activity and give an approximate measure of what frequencies your child can hear and at what volume. The newborn hearing screen is sometimes a quick-and-dirty version of this test that can be done in a few minutes. A detailed ABR can sometimes take several hours and multiple visits to an audiologist.

ABRs are generally the most accurate hearing test for very young children, but they need to be done while a baby is fast asleep and very still. Children over the age of three or four months often have to be sedated for the test to work, although you can sometimes get away with non-sedated ABRs on older babies if you take extra care with their sleep arrangements, keeping them awake and then feeding them at the last minute to really knock them out.

Auditory neuropathy: deafness caused by problems in the transmission of nerve signals along the auditory nerve to the brain. Sometimes associated with fluctuating hearing levels.

Autism, apraxia, dyspraxia, aphasia, auditory processing disorder (APD), and specific language impairment (SLI): Neurological differences that can make it difficult to understand or express language. Deaf kids sometimes have these, which can complicate their language acquisition. Alternatively, hearing kids with one of these differences might use ASL as a primary language or get other "Deaf-style" education or interventions to support them.

bilateral deafness / hearing loss: deafness in both ears.

Booth testing / pure tone testing / audiometry: Big-boy hearing tests where your child sits in a soundproof booth, often on your lap, and reacts to sounds played on speakers or through headphones. There are different strategies for this depending on your kid's age and abilities—little toys your child can look at or play with to indicate they heard the specific tone, but overall it's straightforward "Can you hear this? What about THIS?" stuff.

You will do a lot of these, and if your kid uses technology, this is one way audiologists gauge and tweak devices. They are tricky, though, because they rely on having certain levels of ability and can give ambiguous results.

Conductive deafness / hearing loss: deafness caused by problems in the mechanical chain of sound transmission from the outer ear, through the middle ear, and into the cochlea. Generally, it involves the ear canal, the eardrum, the tiny little ear bones, and so on. Vibrations are not getting through.

Dinner table syndrome: a set of psychiatric symptoms displayed by deaf children who are isolated due to lack of access to language in their families, schools, or peer groups. Dinner table syndrome encompasses both the trauma of isolation and the loss of social skills and incidental learning that can occur when kids don't have access to daily conversations.

Hearing levels: An approximate measure on how deaf your kid is. When written as a medical diagnosis, it's often termed "hearing loss," so you may need to use that when writing in official docs like insurance forms. Keep in mind that even though these are measured in decibels, deafness is not just a volume thing, it's also a detail thing.[1] Speech that is loud enough to hear might still be impossible to understand because of the way particular forms of deafness can blur or scramble sounds. It's like trying to figure out the lyrics to "Louie, Louie"—just blasting the music doesn't actually help.

> **mild deafness / hearing loss**: sounds must be at least 26 to 40 decibels to be heard; speech is usually perceptiblebut can be difficult to understand in noisy environments.
>
> **moderate**: sounds must be at least 41 to 55 decibels to be heard; ordinary speech can be difficult to understand..
>
> **moderate-severe:**[2] sounds must be at least 56 to 70 decibels to be heard; speech can be very difficult or impossible to understand, and only loud sounds might be heard.

---

[1] Audiograms take some of this into account by measuring hearing at different frequencies or pitches, but even that doesn't give you the complete picture.

[2] Depending on whom you ask, "moderately severe" gets rounded up to "severe" in one category from 56–90 dB.

severe: sounds must be at least 71 to 90 decibels to be heard; speech is not possible to understand on its own and only very loud sounds can be heard.
profound: total or near-total deafness; a perfect score.

Language deprivation syndrome: a set of cognitive disabilities caused by a child's lack of access to language in their first three years of life. Language deprivation interferes with later language acquisition and can impair executive function, math and reasoning skills, as well as social function and theory of mind. The damage is neurological—it can be seen in brain imaging scans—and potentially lifelong, depending on its severity.

Microtia and anotia: having small (microtia) or missing ears (anotia) and associated anatomy.

Mixed deafness / hearing loss: deafness caused by a combination of conductive and sensorineural issues.

Newborn hearing screen: The first set of hearing tests your child will get is usually the newborn hearing screen given a day or two after birth in the hospital. These are very rough checks—usually a basic version of an ABR or OAE test. If an issue is found in the hearing screen, more in-depth testing is called for to determine what's up.

Non-verbal: Someone unable to use expressive language. Should not be applied to deaf children who just don't use *spoken* language—if they use ASL, they're verbal.

Otoacoustic emission test (OAE): Another common test that's also sometimes used for newborn screening. Your inner ear makes its own very faint noise in reaction to sound, and an OAE measures this noise. If a kid doesn't have an OAE response, that could mean that their inner ear isn't responding to sound in the typical way, or that there is a blockage somewhere preventing sound from traveling to the inner ear. Compared with ABR, it's fast and doesn't need sedation, but it doesn't give enough information on its own to construct an audiogram.

Prelingual deafness / hearing loss: a child who is born deaf or loses their hearing before they learn their first language (L1). Language deprivation is a major potential obstacle for these children.

postlingual deafness / hearing loss: a child (or adult) who loses their hearing after learning a first language. Postlingually deaf children are generally at lower risk of language deprivation, depending on when they lost their hearing, but face social and communication barriers like dinner table syndrome just like their prelingually deafened peers.

Progressive deafness / hearing loss: a common situation where someone's hearing levels continue to drop over the course of weeks, months, or years.

fluctuating deafness / hearing loss: a less common situation where a person's hearing will vary from day to day. Associated with auditory neuropathy.

Residual hearing: whatever hearing a deaf kid actually has.

Sensorineural deafness / hearing loss: deafness caused by problems in the transmission of nerve signals from the cochlea to the auditory nerve. The electrochemical system of hearing is somehow disrupted.

Single-sided deafness (SSD) or unilateral deafness / hearing loss: deafness in just one ear.

Syndromic deafness: deafness caused by genes that have health impacts on other parts of the body.

non-syndromic deafness: any genetic cause of deafness that's not associated with other health impacts.

Tinnitus: Ringing or other noise in the ears. A very common and annoying symptom of some forms of deafness that can have major impacts on quality of life.

A Field Guide to Professionals

Having a deaf baby will bring an army of medical and educational professionals into your life. Some of them will even be helpful, but it's important to know how few of them actually have any training or familiarity with deaf children, even the ones who absolutely should:

Doctor People

Audiologists (AUDs): Medical specialists who test hearing and help select, adjust, and manage hearing technology like hearing aids or cochlear implants. Since the majority treat adults, it's important to find a pediatric audiologist who's familiar with children's needs.

Although families often look to them for advice on their children's deafness, audiologists are hearing specialists, *but not child or language development specialists*. They typically have no training in deaf education and can carry very outdated beliefs about language acquisition. As the "hearing aid / CI guys," they may have a tendency to overestimate the usefulness of technology.

> **educational audiologists (Ed.Auds):** Like it says on the box, these are audiologists who work for the school district and specialize in children's hearing. Unlike a clinical audiologist, Ed.Auds *should* be familiar with educational issues around deaf kids, and are meant to be the in-house advocates and fix-it folks for helping your child access spoken language in the classroom. Unfortunately, the same caveats about old-fashioned oralist beliefs and poor understanding of language apply to Ed.Auds as well.

Ear, nose, and throat (ENTs), otolaryngologists, and head and neck surgeons: These are all the same person: a surgeon who specializes in face and head plumbing. ENTs are usually the ones looking at your child's anatomy to see if they have physical differences that contribute to their deafness. They'll also do surgeries for things like placing ear tubes, BAHA posts, or cochlear implants. Their skill and experience matter; ask them for their stats.

The typical ENT has only a tiny bit of training, sometimes decades old, on pediatric deafness and usually nothing on childhood language acquisition or education, so nothing they say about your kid's long-term prospects should be taken at all seriously. This includes shit like, "I won't give your child a CI if you're going to teach them sign language."

Genetic counselor: a medical professional who specializes in understanding and explaining the way inherited conditions work in families, and helping you make decisions about your child's health from a medical point of view. Be prepared for a lot of charts!

Neurologist: The brain and nerve people, sometimes encountered if your child's deafness is the result of a syndrome or injury that affects the brain. Because some symptoms of pediatric deafness overlap or mask other neurological conditions, it can be important to coordinate care with a specialist who's savvy to deafness and how it can impact other diagnoses.

neuropsychologist: A specialist in the interactions between the brain and behavior. If you have a child with a neurological injury or a syndrome that impacts their nervous system, you may work with a neuropsych.

Occupational therapists (OTs): A therapist that works with children on their fine motor coordination, usually daily tasks you use your hands for: feeding and dressing yourself, using sign language, drawing, and writing, and so on. Some forms of syndromic deafness come with fine motor disabilities, but deaf children are just as likely as hearing children to have unrelated fine motor issues.

Pediatricians (Peds), general practitioners and family physicians (GPs): The typical Ped or GP has nearly zero training in pediatric deafness and absolutely no training in childhood language acquisition or deaf education. So whatever else they might know, when it comes to your kid's language or schooling, their opinion basically doesn't matter, unless you need them as a gateway referral to more specialized services. In that case, you'll need to say "Yes, Doctor" before going back to ignoring them.

Physical therapists (PTs): A therapist that works with gross motor coordination—crawling, standing and walking, climbing stairs, jumping on the bed, and assorted horseplay. It's particularly common for kids with some forms of deafness to have disruptions in their inner ear, creating challenges around balance, but there are many reasons your child may need PT services.

Speech-language pathologists (SLPs): Therapists who work with both speech and language (and swallowing, too). You should always have an SLP monitoring your baby's language acquisition in whatever languages they use—ASL, English, or another home language—and making sure both their understanding and their ability to express language are on track. If there are problems with either expressive or receptive language, it's the SLP who is called in as the primary therapist. My kid actually has two SLPs: one monitors and works on his English-language skills, and another works on his ASL.

Along with teachers of the deaf and Deaf mentors, SLPs are some of the most important professionals your child will have contact with. A good SLP is a treasure; a bad one can set your child's language development back *years*. Be wary of SLPs who discourage using sign language or who focus narrowly on speech and hearing when your child's basic language milestones aren't being met. SLPs who specialize in Listening and Spoken Language (LSL) or Auditory-Verbal Therapy (AVT) are especially prone to this—LSL / AVT is not any better supported by peer-reviewed research than "vanilla" speech-language therapy, but LSL-certified professionals are certified through AG Bell, which has a horrible track record of prioritizing speech over language acquisition and creating language deprivation in deaf children.

Teacher People

Deaf educational advocate: A trained professional who can advise you on your and your child's educational rights under state and federal law. Advocates are sometimes lawyers, but are always familiar with the processes of IFSP, IEP, and 504 planning, and can attend meetings with you, help you draft plans or letters to your district, and generally assist you in getting your child the education they are guaranteed under IDEA. A solid advocate is a must-have when dealing with a difficult school district.

Deaf mentor or Deaf coach: Trained Deaf professionals who visit families to help with all aspects of raising a deaf kid. They act as role models and language models for deaf children and their siblings and support parents and children with ASL language acquisition, but are also available to answer questions about educational choices, access at local events and venues, and the local Deaf community. For hearing parents, Deaf mentors are often the first Deaf people you'll get to know socially. Get 'em if you can!

General education teacher (GenEd): Your run-of-the-mill public school teacher. May be awesome in many ways, but when dealing with a young deaf child, probably in over their head.

Local educational agency (LEA): This term has two meanings: LEAs are both the *organization* that administers early intervention or special education to your child (aka "the district") and they're the *person* who represents your local educational agency at your IFSP and IEP meeting. They can be administrators, teachers, or other professionals, and chances are they have no clue about childhood deafness.

Special education teacher (SpEd): Teachers trained in educating kids with a wide array of disabilities, but usually not specifically deafness. May be awesome in many ways, but when dealing with a young deaf child, probably in over their head.

Teachers of the deaf (ToDs): Teachers who have studied deaf child development, language acquisition, and other essential educational issues for deaf kids. ToDs can work in schools full-time or visit children in schools or at home as itinerant teachers. ToDs are often the folks assessing your child's language development. Their methods and training can vary widely and will tend to track deaf educational philosophies: Bilingual-Bicultural, Total Communication, Listening and Spoken Language. Like SLPs, ToDs are critical to your child's long-term success or failure, so in the case of a hearing ToD trying to support a child in ASL, you need to be sure they actually have the skills to do so.

Index

504 plans   26, 150–2, 172–4, 205, 207

AAC. *See* augmentative and alternative communication
ABI. *See* hearing devices, auditory brainstem implant
ABR. *See* hearing test, auditory brainstem response
ADA. *See* Americans with Disabilities Act
AEP. *See* hearing test, auditory evoked potential
American Sign Language   9, 10, 16, 23–4
   alphabet, ABCs   32
   classes and courses   21–3
   classifiers   32–3, 95
   games   92–4
   media for children   77
   signing with your baby   30–6
   sign names   39–42
   storytelling, poetry, rhythms & rhymes   75–7
Americans with Disabilities Act   137–8, 207–8
anotia. *See* microtia and anotia
AOT. *See* oralism, auditory-oral training
ASL. *See* American Sign Language
AuD. *See* audiologist
audiogram   217–19
   cookie bite, reverse cookie bite   257
   flat deafness   256
   sloping, reverse slope   256
   speech banana   218–19, 256
audiologist   7, 17, 26, 45, 67, 96, 122, 175, 206, 217–19, 227–8, 241, 256, 261
   educational   206, 261
audiology. *See* hearing test
audism   201, 253
auditory brainstem response, auditory evoked potential. *See* hearing test, auditory brainstem response
auditory neuropathy   257, 260
auditory oral training. *See* oralism, auditory-oral training
auditory verbal training. *See* oralism, auditory-verbal training
augmentative and alternative communication   20, 148–9
autism, the autism spectrum   3, 225–6, 257
AVT. *See* oralism, auditory-verbal training

babbling   35
Baby Signs, baby sign language   12–13
babysitters. *See* childcare
bad professionals   117, 174–84, 206–7
   firing and management   117, 174–84, 206–7
   red flags   12, 181–2, 197
   red lines   182–4
BAHA. *See* hearing devices, bone anchored hearing aid
Bathing   46
BiBi. *See* education, Bilingual-Bicultural
bilateral deafness   257
bilingualism   194–7, 204
blind. *See* Deafblind
bone anchored hearing aids. *See* hearing devices, bone anchored hearing aids

captions, closed captions   50, 67, 99
car mirrors   51
carriers and backpacks   51
car seats   50–2
CDI. *See* interpreters, certified Deaf interpreter
childcare   184–90
child of Deaf adults   30, 54, 56, 57, 188, 253
CI. *See* hearing devices, cochlear implant
clothes   48, 61, 64–5
CMV. *See* cytomegalovirus
cochlear implants. *See* hearing devices, cochlear implant
CODA. *See* child of Deaf adults
conductive deafness   226, 229, 231, 258
cytomegalovirus   220, 222

deaf   1, 10, 254
Deaf   21, 24, 254
Deaf +, Deaf Plus. *See* Deaf Disabled
DeafBlind, Deafblind, deafblind   20, 55, 149, 167, 221, 255
Deaf culture   37–42, 108–15, 125–6, 132–3, 136–7, 195–6
Deaf Disabled   20, 133, 148, 157, 161–2, 173, 192–3, 203, 219–21, 223–4, 254–5
deaf gain   255
Deaf mentors, Deaf coaches   21, 22, 24–5, 90, 155, 193, 223, 263
Deaf President Now (DPN)   137
deaf school. *See* education, schools for the deaf
deaf services agency   20–22, 26, 152, 155, 163, 193
diagnosis, identification, causes of deafness   25, 149, 160, 217–18
dinner table syndrome   66, 79–86, 98–101, 196, 258
doctors   3, 7, 17, 25, 30, 84, 122, 149, 160, 174, 212–27, 234, 235, 238–9, 261
    ear nose & throat, otolaryngologists, head & neck surgeons   261
    general practitioner (GP)   262

neurologist   262
neuropsychologist   262
pediatrician   262

early childhood education   185–6, 188
Early Intervention   21, 23–7, 136, 139, 149–84, 218
    referral   25–6, 160, 218 (*see also* individual educational plan and individual family service plan)
ECE. *See* early childhood education
EdAuD. *See* audiologist, educational
education   3, 10–17, 21–4, 121–211
    Bilingual-Bicultural   136, 195–6
    deaf educational philosophies   194–9
    history of deaf education   123–40
    mainstream schools, mainstreaming   200–10
    oral deaf education   198–9
    preschools & daycares   184–94, 196, 198
    schools for the deaf   21, 124–39
    Total Communication   132, 134, 136, 143, 197–8, 203 (*see also* sign language education for parents, childcare)
emotional health
    parents   89–90, 94–8, 247–8, 251 (*see also* language deprivation, dinner table syndrome
    siblings and children   87–92
eugenics   123, 126–31, 140

family   47, 79–107
    abusive   103–7, 116–17
    extended family   98–104
    family events & holidays   98–102
    nuts (*see* abusive)
    parenting   7–27, 30–77, 79–98
        dads   54, 95–7
        maintenance sex   97–8
        moms   54, 94–7
    siblings   86–92, 155, 188, 254
family background   108–19

Asian American and Pacific
   Islander   109–10, 163
Black, African-American   110–11,
   163
Latine, Latino, and Hispanic
   111–12, 163
Native American and First
   Nations   113, 163 (*see also*
   religion)
FAPE. *See* free and appropriate public
   education
FAQ. *See* frequently asked questions
first language   8–9, 19, 140–2
fluctuating deafness/hearing loss   218,
   257, 260
food
   feeding   45–6
   grocery store, supermarket   52–3
   mealtimes   37, 49, 80 (*see also*
      American Sign Language, games)
free and appropriate public
   education   208–10
frequently asked questions   10–27
   cochlear implants   232–5
   hearing aid, CROS, and BAHA
      240–2
   interpreters   214–16
   smart questions   114
   stupid questions   99, 248

Gallaudet University   124, 126, 131, 132,
   137, 139
gender. *See* parenting
GenEd. *See* teacher, general education
genetics   91–2, 220–1, 224–5, 260
   gene therapy   18, 222
   genetic councilor   261 (*see also* non-
      genetic causes of deafness)
   genetic testing   220–1, 224–5

HA. *See* hearing devices, hearing aids
hard of hearing   1, 3, 7, 18–19, 181, 255
hearing aids. *See* hearing devices, hearing
   aids
hearing devices

auditory brainstem implants   231
   at the beach or pool   60–1
   bone anchored hearing aids   17, 44–5,
      52, 228–30, 240–4
   in the car   52–3
   cochlear implants   17, 44–5, 91–2,
      134–6, 228, 230–40, 243–4
   in the crib   44–5
   CROS, BICROS, cross systems
      44–5, 228, 230, 240–4
   hearing aids   17, 44–5, 134–6, 228,
      229, 240–4
   middle ear implants   231
   at the playground   54–5
   in snow and cold   65
   in the wilderness   63
hearing levels   256, 258
   mild   18–19, 258
   moderate   18–19, 258
   moderate-severe   258
   profound   259
   severe   258
hearing tests
   auditory brainstem response, auditory
      evoked potential   138, 217–18,
      257, 259
   booth testing, audiometry, pure tone
      testing   17–19, 96, 258
   otoacoustic emission   259
HH/HoH. *See* hard of hearing
home improvement and accessibility   49
   deaf doorbells, visual doorbells   49
   deaf smoke detectors, visual smoke
      detectors   49
   mirrors   49

IDEA. *See* Individuals with Disabilities
   Education Act
IEP. *See* individual educational plan
IFSP. *See* individual family service plan
individual educational plan   26, 27,
   94, 96, 122, 133, 139, 150–60,
   182, 205
individual family service plan   26, 27, 94,
   122, 139, 150–60, 182, 205

assessments, IEP and IFSP   153, 165–6, 170–1
goals, IEP and IFSP   153, 171–2
interpreters, IEP and IFSP   207–8
meetings, IEP and IFSP   151–60
school placement, IEP and IFSP   154, 164–5, 208–10
services, IEP and IFSP   153, 166–71
timeline, IFSP   160–1
transition meeting, IEP   161, 164–5
Individuals with Disabilities Education Act   133, 136, 139, 149–74, 180, 181, 203, 207–10, 263
interpreters   61, 66–7, 77, 84–6, 100–1, 163
certified Deaf interpreter   216
church interpreters   115
educational interpreters   204–8
hiring and firing   174–84, 211–16
medical interpreters   212–13, 216
Video Relay Interpreting   216

kitchen table games. *See* American Sign Language, games

L1. *See* first language
language deprivation syndrome, language deprivation   8, 12, 16–19, 68, 92, 126, 136, 138, 141, 144, 146, 149, 158, 187, 192, 195–9, 239, 259
Language Equality and Acquisition for Deaf Kids   139
LEAD-K milestones   35, 36, 152
language neglect. *See* dinner table syndrome
language window   8, 18, 122, 136, 194
late deafened   255
LEA. *See* local educational agency or local educational agent
LEAD-K. *See* Language Equality and Acquisition for Deaf Kids
least restrictive environment   164, 208–10
Ling-6 sounds   158, 207, 218–19
linguicism   226, 253

lip reading. *See* speechreading
listening and spoken language. *See* oralism, listening and spoken language
literacy. *See* reading
literacy. *See* reading
local educational agency (school district)   24, 149–83, 187, 198, 200–1, 203, 207–10
local educational agent (district representative)   151, 153, 156, 159, 163, 168, 171, 176–83, 264
LRE. *See* least restrictive environment
LSL. *See* oralism, listening and spoken language

mainstreaming. *See* education, mainstream schools
MEI. *See* hearing devices, middle ear implant
microtia and anotia   256, 259
mixed deafness   226, 259

name signs. *See* American Sign Language, sign names
nanny. *See* childcare
National Technical Institute for the Deaf   133
neuropsychologist   156, 262
non-genetic causes of deafness   219, 222–4
NTID. *See* National Technical Institute for the Deaf
nursery rhymes. *See* American Sign Language, storytelling, poetry, rhythms & rhymes

OAE. *See* hearing tests, otoacoustic emission
oralism   126–38
auditory-oral training   135, 199
auditory-verbal training   16, 135, 162, 263
listening and spoken language   16, 135, 198–9

potty training and diapers   7, 46
progressive deafness or hearing loss   2, 18–19, 218, 220, 236, 255
prosthetics. *See* hearing devices

quick start guides
    deaf baby quick start   7–27
    hearing devices quick start   227–32
    IFSP and IEP quick start   152–60

race. *See* family background
racism   121, 163. *See also* eugenics
reading   67–74
Rehabilitation Act of (1973)   133, 151, 172, 200
relatives. *See* family
religion   115–19
    faith healing   116–17
    proselytizers and missionaries   117
    religious denominations   117–19
        atheism   119
        Catholic church   118
        Episcopal church   117
        Islam   119
        Judaism   118–19
        Latter-Day Saints (LDS)   118
        Orthodox church   118
        other Christian denominations   118
        paganism   119
residual hearing   9, 16, 18–19, 36, 44, 46, 47, 67, 161–2, 218, 226, 229–31, 234, 240–1, 260

SEE. *See* sign systems, Signed Exact English
sensorineural deafness   218, 256, 260
sex   97–98
sign language, signed language   3, 9–11, 16, 20–4, 30–6
    American Sign Language (ASL) (*see* American Sign Language)
    Australian Sign Language (Auslan)   11, 74
    Black American Sign Language (BASL)   110–11, 131
    British Sign Language (BSL)   75
    French Sign Language, *Langue des Signes Française* (LSF)   11, 124
    Japanese Sign Language (JSL)   115
    Mexican Sign Langage *Lengua de Señas Mexicana (LSM)*   11, 112, 115
natural languages   7, 11, 141–2, 149, 197
ProTactile   20, 221, 255
tactile ASL (TASL)   20
sign systems   11–14, 140–8, 194–5, 197–8
    Conceptually Accurate Signed English (CASE)   142
    Cued Speech (CS), Cued English   11, 146–7
    Makaton   11, 148
    Manually Coded English (MCE)   11, 142
    Pidgin Signed English (PSE), contact sign   145–6
    Signed Exact English (SEE)   11, 21, 68, 132, 137, 142–5
    Sign English (SE)   142
    Sign Supported English (SSE)   11, 147
SimCom. *See* simultaneous communication
simultaneous communication   33–34, 134, 143, 147, 197–8, 213
single-sided deafness   18, 211, 230, 241, 260
sleep   42–5
    sleep training   42
    soothing   44
SLP. *See* speech-language pathology
special education   25, 26, 134, 139, 150, 163, 187, 200, 203. *See also* individual educational plan
SpEd. *See* special education teacher
SpEd. *See* teacher, special education
speech   14–15, 126, 129–31, 176, 198–9, 235, 238–42
    speech banana (*see* audiogram)
    speech therapy   14–16, 131
speech-language pathology, pathologist   8, 14, 35, 114, 161, 174–84, 196, 262–3

speechreading 15–16, 126, 135, 199
SSD. *See* single-sided deafness
strollers and bassinets 51
subtitles. *See* captions
syndromic deafness 220–1, 260
    non-syndromic deafness 220–1, 260

TC. *See* education, Total Communication
teacher
    general education 200–3, 205, 264
    itinerant teacher of the deaf 186, 198, 206
    special education 203, 205, 264
    teacher of the deaf 8, 35, 114, 161, 174–84, 196, 200–1, 206–7, 264
terps. *See* interpreters

therapists
    occupational 151, 262
    physical 151, 262
    psychiatric, psychologists 30, 89–90, 165, 223, 227
tinnitus 227
ToD. *See* teacher, teacher of the deaf
toys 47–8
trauma. *See* emotional health

unilateral deafness. *See* single-sided deafness

video relay interpreting 212, 216
visual baby 43, 61
VRI. *See under* interpreters, video relay interpreting

About the Author

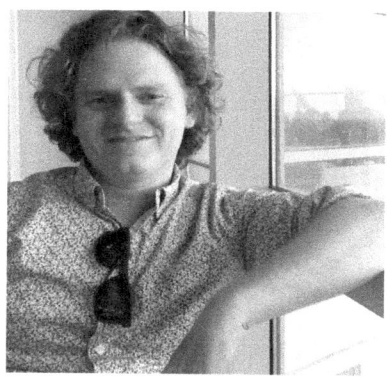

Will Fertman is a father and writer. He lives with his family in Northern California. Read more of his work, and find parenting resources for deaf children, at willfertman.com.